CW00693469

The Herb Companion

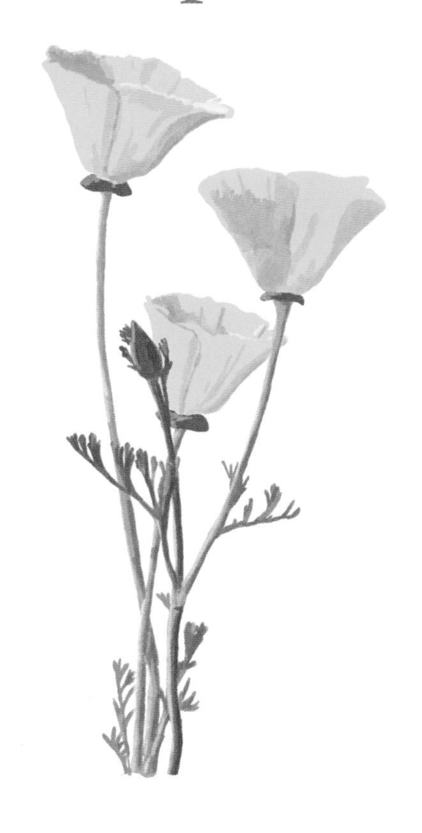

APPLE

First published in the UK in 2016 by
APPLE PRESS
74-77 White Lion Street
London N1 9PF
United Kingdom

www.apple-press.com

This book was designed, conceived and produced by
Quantum Books Ltd
6 Blundell Street
London N7 9BH
United Kingdom

Publisher: Kerry Enzor
Project Editor: Alison Candlin
Art Editor: Louise Turpin
Illustration: Andrew Pinder
Cover Design: Rupert Gowar-Cliffe and Tokiko Morishima
Production Manager: Zarni Win

ISBN 978-1-84543-649-0

Toppan Leefung Printers Limited, printed in China

2 4 6 8 10 9 7 5 3 1

QUMTHC1

The material in this book has previously appeared as *The Herb Companion*, by Marcus A. Webb, published in 2000 by Quintet Publishing Ltd.

The Herb Companion

The Essential Guide to Using Herbs for Your Health and Well-being

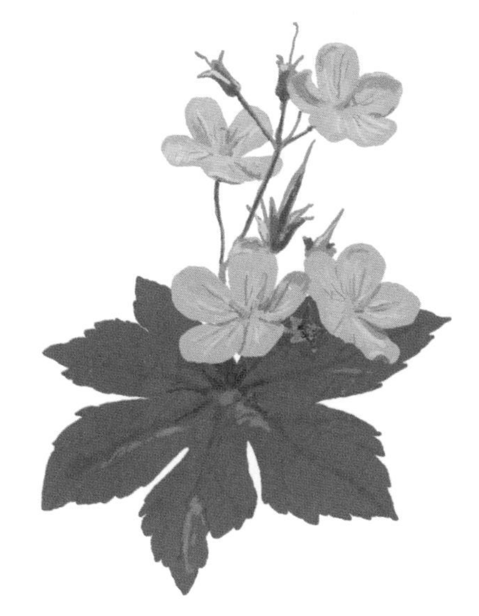

Edited by Alison Candlin

APPLE

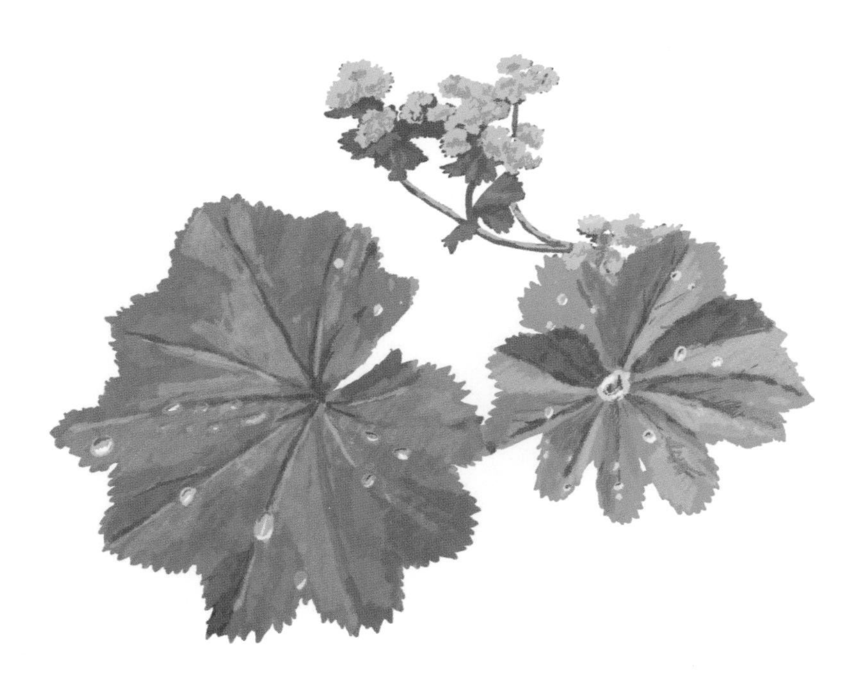

Contents

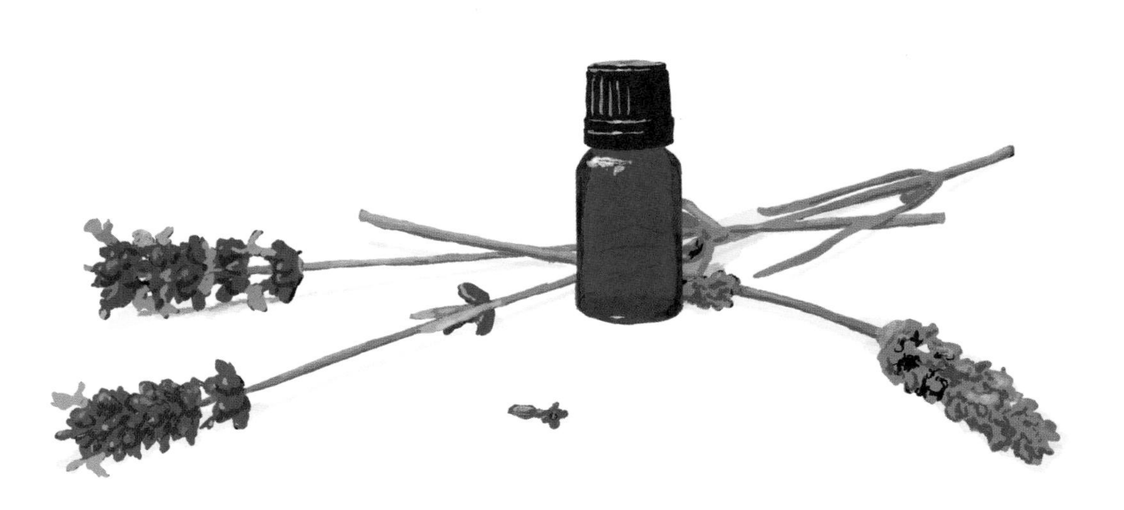

List of Herbs by Common Name

Introduction

Herbs can do far more for you than just garnish a finished dish. The use of herbs for the promotion of health can be dated back to the days of Hippocrates, who compiled a *materia medica* (a book containing information on herbs and their prescription) of more than 400 medicinal herbs during his lifetime (c. 460–370 B.C.). The works he left behind were soon built upon. The Greek philosopher Aristotle (c. 372–287 B.C.) wrote his monumental 10-volume compendium called *The History of Plants*, making him one of the most important contributors to our knowledge of botanical science.

The first illustrated book on herbal preparations was written by the English herbalist and surgeon John Gerard. *The Herball*, or *Generall Historie of Plantes*, was published in 1597 and gave comprehensive details of each plant, including its origin, history, uses, methods of planting and the type of soil needed for each different species. By 1785 herbs were being used for the treatment of many problems, one of which pushed forwards the science of pharmacology dramatically. An English physician, William Withering, discovered that dropsy (heart failure) could be successfully treated with an extract of foxglove (*Digitalis*). This extract is still used to the present day in the form of the drug Digoxin.

Growing Herbs

Herbs are not difficult to grow, and great satisfaction can be gained from cultivating an herb garden or even growing just a pot of herbs. Plant herbs outside if there is no risk of them being damaged by excessive heat or cold. Most herbs enjoy a sunny location, but chives, feverfew, horseradish, lemon balm, mint, comfrey, ginger, angelica and parsley are best planted in a shady place. Many herbs will do well indoors if you don't have space in your garden, though this will limit your growing capabilities. The commonly used culinary and medicinal herbs are all worth considering when choosing what to grow.

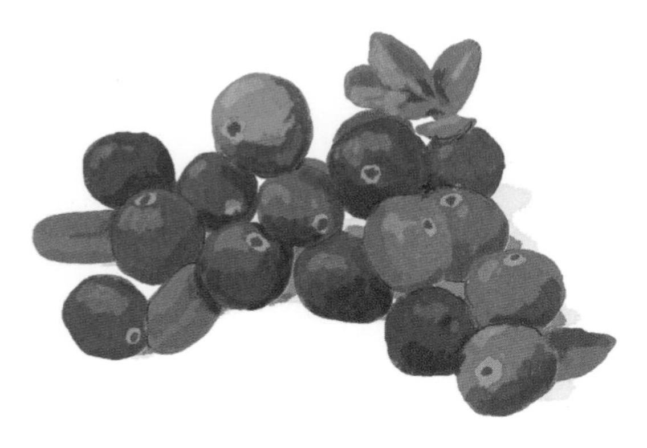

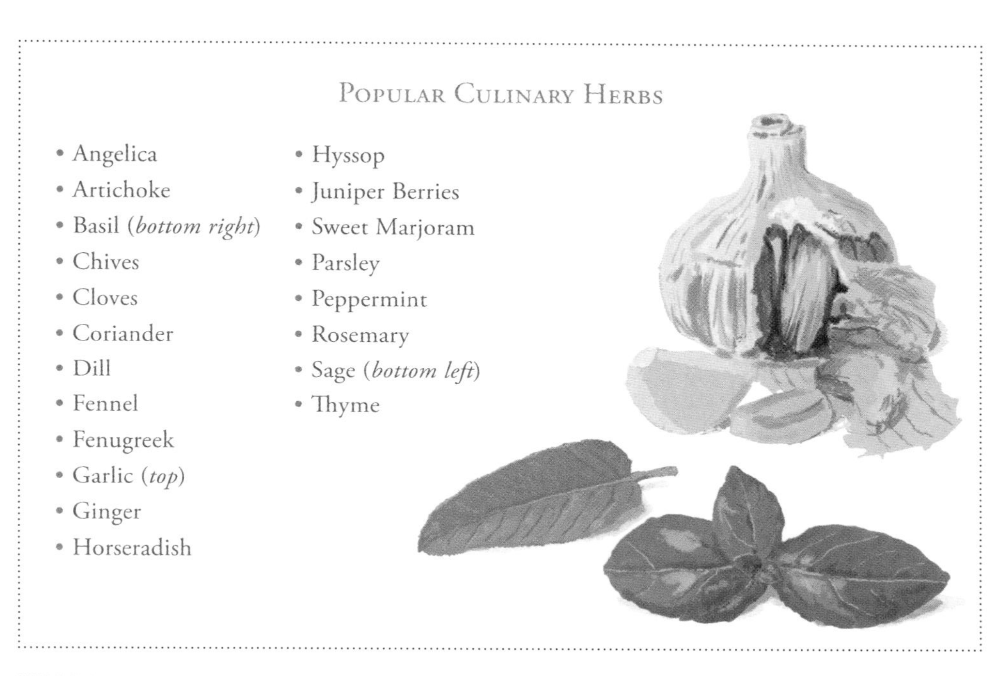

Popular Culinary Herbs

- Angelica
- Artichoke
- Basil (*bottom right*)
- Chives
- Cloves
- Coriander
- Dill
- Fennel
- Fenugreek
- Garlic (*top*)
- Ginger
- Horseradish
- Hyssop
- Juniper Berries
- Sweet Marjoram
- Parsley
- Peppermint
- Rosemary
- Sage (*bottom left*)
- Thyme

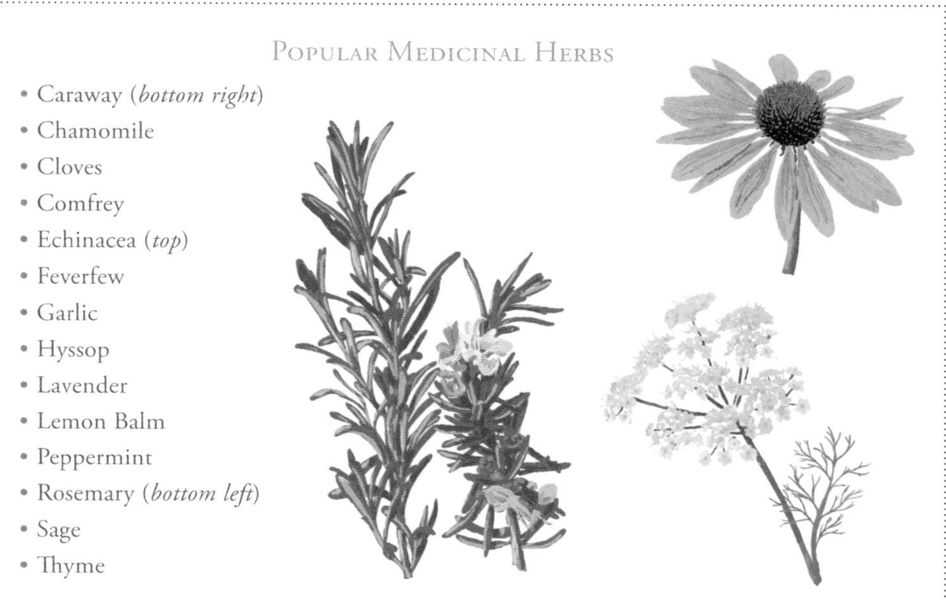

Popular Medicinal Herbs

- Caraway (*bottom right*)
- Chamomile
- Cloves
- Comfrey
- Echinacea (*top*)
- Feverfew
- Garlic
- Hyssop
- Lavender
- Lemon Balm
- Peppermint
- Rosemary (*bottom left*)
- Sage
- Thyme

Harvesting Herbs

Picking herbs tends to encourage new growth and stimulates the healthy development of the plant. When picking the flowers it is best to take the bud just before it opens up, as most herbs reach their optimal flavour just prior to flowering. Perennial herbs can yield two or three good crops during their growing seasons, but it is best to give them one year to get established before harvesting. When collecting from perennials, it is important not to cut into the woody growth. For annuals it is possible to cut the crop to 10cm (4in) from the soil twice during the growing season with a final harvesting just before the first frost.

If you wish to collect the seeds, wait until the seedpods change colour. To confirm if they are ready, just give the pods a tap; if seeds fall out, they are ready to be gathered. If you wish to collect the roots or rhizomes for use, wait until the above-ground stems and leaves have died back and the plant goes into a dormant state, and then dig up the underground structures.

Making Remedies

Infusions and Decoctions

Infusions are made by adding boiling water to the delicate parts of the herb – the flowers, leaves and seeds. An infusion is normally made from a single herb, and it should never consist of more than three herbs. For the hardy parts of a plant – the wood, bark and stems – a decoction is used to extract the active agents from this tough material.

The same quantities are used as for an infusion, but the water and herbs are brought to a boil from cold, then simmered for 20 minutes before they are strained and drunk. Infusion and decoction preparations are best taken the day they are made, but they can be kept in the fridge for about 24 hours.

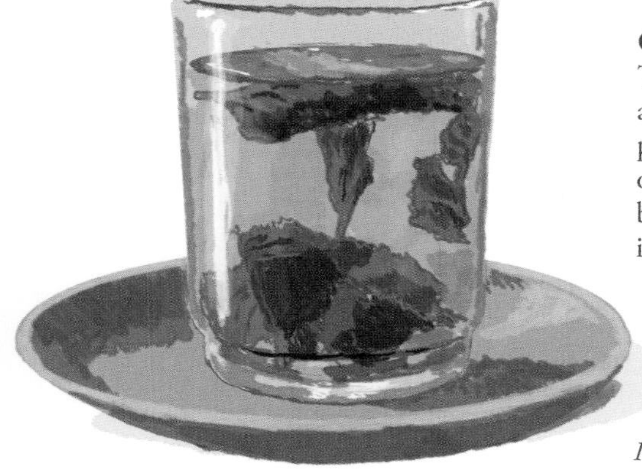

Peppermint tea

Tinctures

To make a tincture, the herbs (any part can be used) are steeped for just over two weeks in an alcohol and water mixture. The process extracts the active agents from the plant matter, while the alcohol content of the mixture preserves the tincture for about two years from the date of manufacture. After about two weeks, press out the mixture to obtain the final tincture. Seal in an airtight container and use as needed.

It is best to make tinctures of single herbs and only combine them with other tinctures when needed. Your local pharmacy can supply you with the alcohol needed for the extraction process. Commercial tinctures use ethyl alcohol but you can make tinctures at home using vodka (37.5%). Dilute 750ml (1¼ pints) vodka with 2½ tablespoons water and use this mixture to steep the herbs in.

Oils

The extraction of oils from plant material is a complex process and it is probably best to purchase commercially produced essential oils. Essential oils tend to evaporate when brought into contact with the air, so it is vitally important to keep the lids on bottles of essential oils firmly closed to preserve the aroma. When mixing oils for use in massage, keep the

Evening primrose oil

combinations simple, and limit yourself to no more than four oils in any one remedy. It is perfectly acceptable to use a single oil, and this may actually exert a more powerful effect than if it were combined with others.

Oils in Massage

Oils for use in massage have been classified according to the part of the plant from which they have been extracted. Oils derived from the flowers are termed the top notes and carry the presenting aroma that is first noticed; those from the leaves are called the middle notes and have a more therapeutic action; oils from the wood and roots are known as the base notes, as they provide a 'fixing' characteristic to a blend since they have a more long-lasting aroma. A formula with a balanced blend of oils, therefore, carries all of these notes.

The oil into which the essential oils are mixed is referred to as the carrier, or base oil and is commonly grapeseed or almond oil. Others, such as wheatgerm or avocado oil, can be used, but these are normally reserved for very dry skin types because of the nutritive nature of the oil.

Poultices and Compresses

The best method of making a poultice is to use the fresh leaves, stems and roots. Chop and crush the material into a paste, adding water as needed to form a good consistency. A short whizz in a blender or food processor can speed up the process. The final processed herb can be either applied directly to the skin or placed between two thin layers of gauze and bound firmly to the area. The poultice can be bearably hot or cold, but the best method of keeping it active is to place a hot water bottle over the gauze for about 30 minutes. This can be repeated every two to three hours as needed.

Medicinal Uses

It is important to keep in mind that plant extracts can be very toxic as well as beneficial to health. Just because they are natural does not mean they are safe; some of the most powerful poisons are obtained from plants. In order to make the use of herbal medicine safe and effective, you need to know how much and how often to take an extract. Just as a medicine bottle from the pharmacy tells you how much aspirin is in each tablet, so a bottle of herbal medicine should tell you how much active agent is contained in it. This not only safeguards against overdosage, but it also reassures you that you are taking a good-quality extract.

Medicine Cabinet Staples

There are a number of essential herbs that are best kept as tinctures or ready-made tablets or capsules so that they are always ready for instant use. Tinctures of echinacea (*Echinacea purpura*) and valerian (*Valeriana officinalis*) are always good to have in store, as well as preparations of licorice (*Glycyrrhiza glabra*), Korean ginseng (*Panax ginseng*) and cranberry (*Vaccinium macrocarpon*).

CAUTIONARY NOTE:

At all times it is recommended that you consult a health-care professional before embarking on a programme of self-treatment. Herbal medicines are effective and safe when used in the correct circumstances. This book has been written to educate, and every effort has been made to make the book as accurate and as informative as possible, but the advice contained within is no replacement for professional guidance.

Directory of Herbs

Herbs add flavour and depth to cooking and have myriad uses in cosmetic creams and lotions or herbal remedies for a wide range of ailments and conditions. These pages list both common and lesser-known herbs – arranged alphabetically by their botanical name – showing the different forms in which they are available and explaining their uses in cooking and traditional medicine. The list of herbs on pages 6–7 will help you to find a particular herb if you know it only by its common name. Always consult a qualified medical practitioner before treating ailments yourself at home.

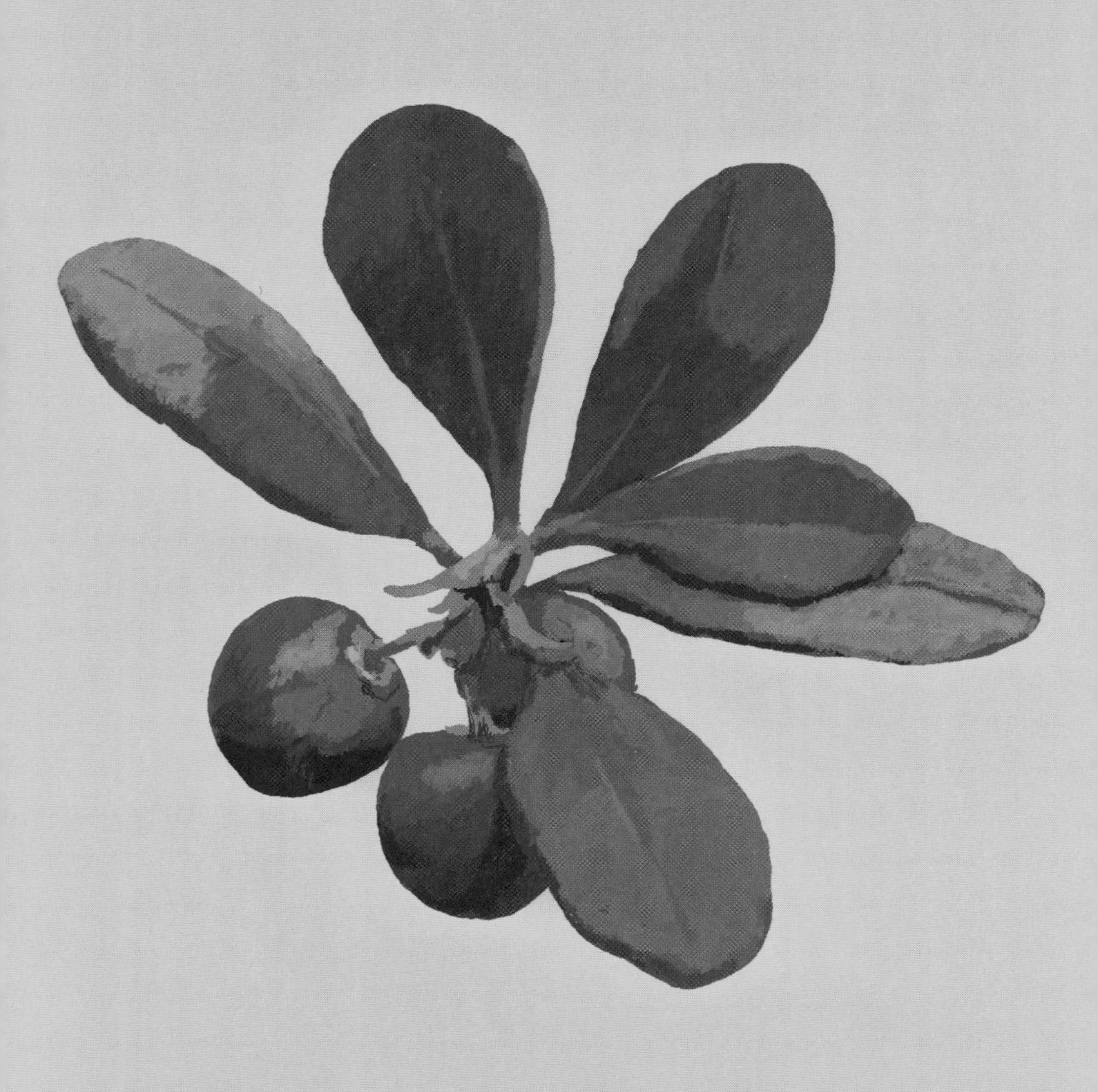

Yarrow
Achillea millefolium

The Latin name for this plant is believed to come from the Greek hero Achilles. It is said that he used it to heal his soldiers' wounds during the Trojan War. Taken internally, this herb is used to stimulate the circulatory system and help to reduce blood pressure.

Origins & Characteristics
Yarrow has a diaphoretic action, so it is helpful in reducing fevers brought about by colds and flu. It also has antiseptic and anti-inflammatory properties, so it is used to control excessive bleeding and helps reduce diarrhoea and dysentery. This herb can be used to relieve indigestion, flatulence and dyspepsia.

Externally, yarrow is used to help heal minor wounds and for cleansing and toning the skin.

Parts Used
Leaves and flowers

Dosage
As a tea, add about 2 teaspoons of herbs to 600ml (1 pint) of boiling water and infuse for 5 minutes.

For external application use yarrow as a poultice for minor cuts and scrapes.

Potential Benefits
- Stimulates the circulatory system
- Helps reduce blood pressure
- Helps to reduce fevers
- Has antiseptic properties
- Has anti-inflammatory properties
- Can reduce diarrhoea
- Can relieve indigestion

Cosmetic Uses
Flowers can be used in creams and lotions to cleanse the skin. Yarrow can also be used in skin tonics as an astringent treatment for oily skin.

Culinary Uses
The fresh young leaves are used in salads.

Caution
Do not use yarrow for long periods as it may cause skin irritation. Avoid during pregnancy.

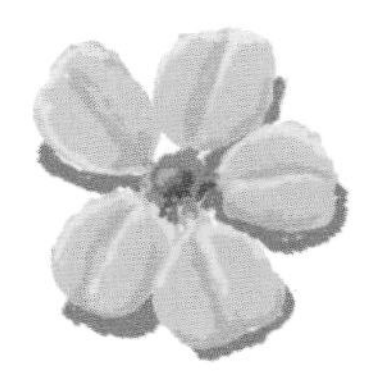

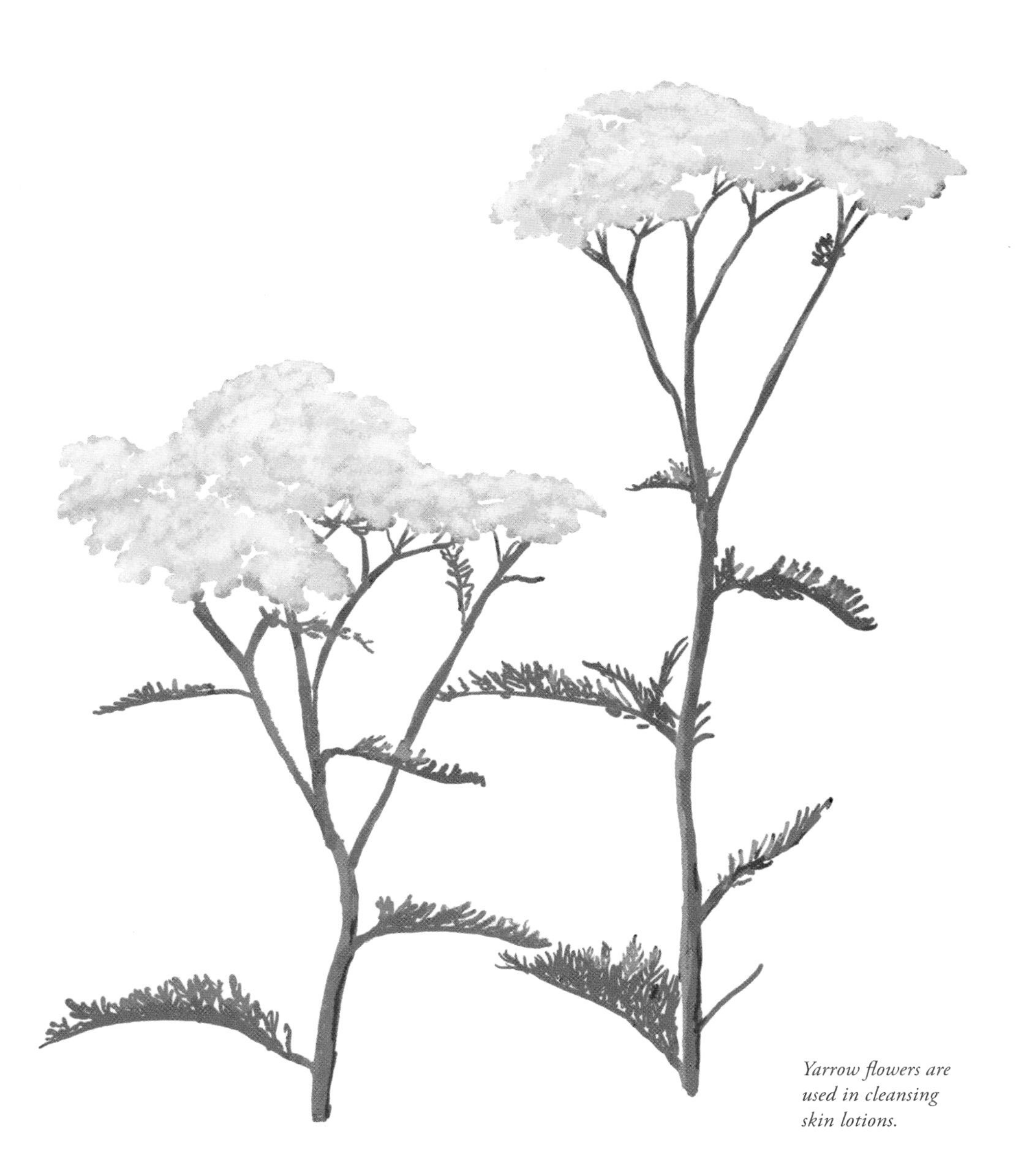

Yarrow flowers are used in cleansing skin lotions.

Sweet Flag
Acorus calamus

This herb has both medicinal and culinary uses. A sweet treat made from this plant is produced by crystallizing tender slices of the roots (rhizomes). The roots contain volatile oils that have profound antibiotic actions.

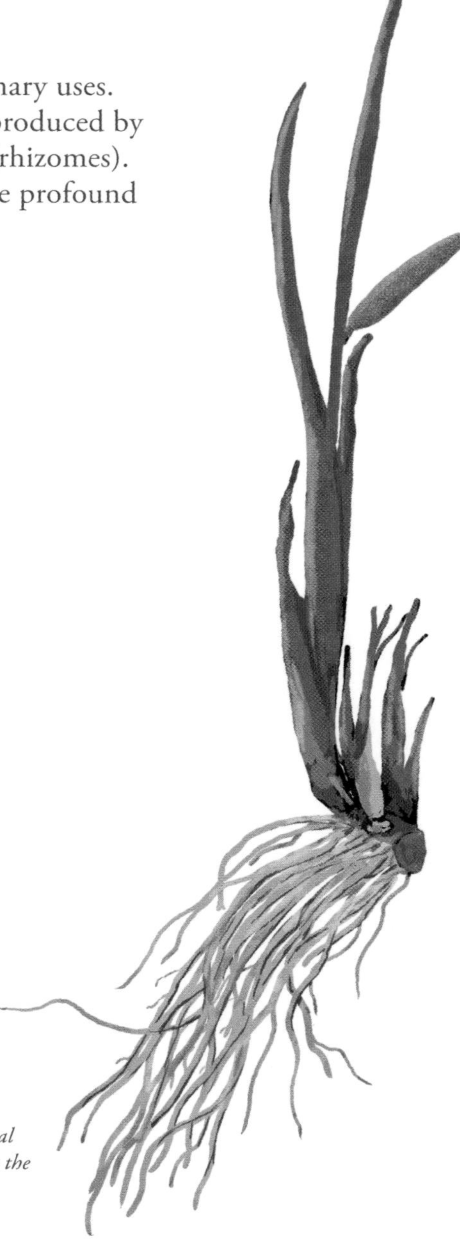

Origins & Characteristics
Taken internally, sweet flag can be very useful in the stimulation of digestion and as a remedy for bronchitis and sinus congestion. As an external application, it can be used to relieve rheumatic joint and muscle pains. It is also a carminative agent and can reduce muscular spasms that are associated with nerve pains.

Parts Used
Roots, rhizomes and oil extract

Dosage
As a liquid tincture, take 20 drops twice daily before eating. For external application, use as a compress for joint and muscle pain.

Potential Benefits
- Helps bronchitis
- Reduces sinus congestion
- Stimulates digestion
- Eases joint and muscle pains
- May help in neuralgia

Culinary Uses
Used to make sweets.

The active medicinal part of sweet flag is the roots, or rhizomes.

Horse Chestnut
Aesculus hippocastanum

The leaves of this tree leave a horseshoe-shaped scar behind on the twig as they fall off, but it is named horse chestnut because the fruits were used as fodder for cattle and horses. Herbal medicine has found a number of applications for this herb, particularly as a remedy for treating or easing problems with the circulation.

Origins & Characteristics

When taken internally, horse chestnut has a mild diuretic activity and an anti-inflammatory effect. This herb can improve the flow and exchange of tissue fluids in the body and reduce swelling associated with poor circulation. Therefore, the congestion that occurs in cases of varicose veins can be relieved by regular use of an extract of horse chestnut.

Its value in circulatory problems can be seen by the benefit reported by those who have suffered a stroke or suffer from erythema or other conditions associated with poor circulation – it promotes the flow of oxygenated blood to every area of the body.

Parts Used

Bark and seeds

Dosage

As a liquid tincture, take 15–20 drops twice daily. For external application, apply as a cream directly to varicose veins.

Potential Benefits

- Acts as a mild diuretic
- Regulates circulation
- Reduces tissue inflammation
- Eases varicose vein symptoms
- Promotes flow of oxygenated blood to all areas of the body

Cosmetic Uses

May be used in a lotion to improve the skin's circulation.

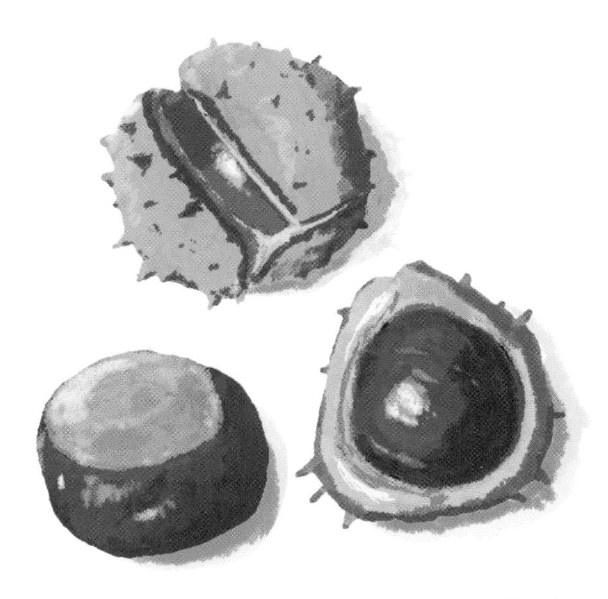

Conkers contain healing properties for the circulation.

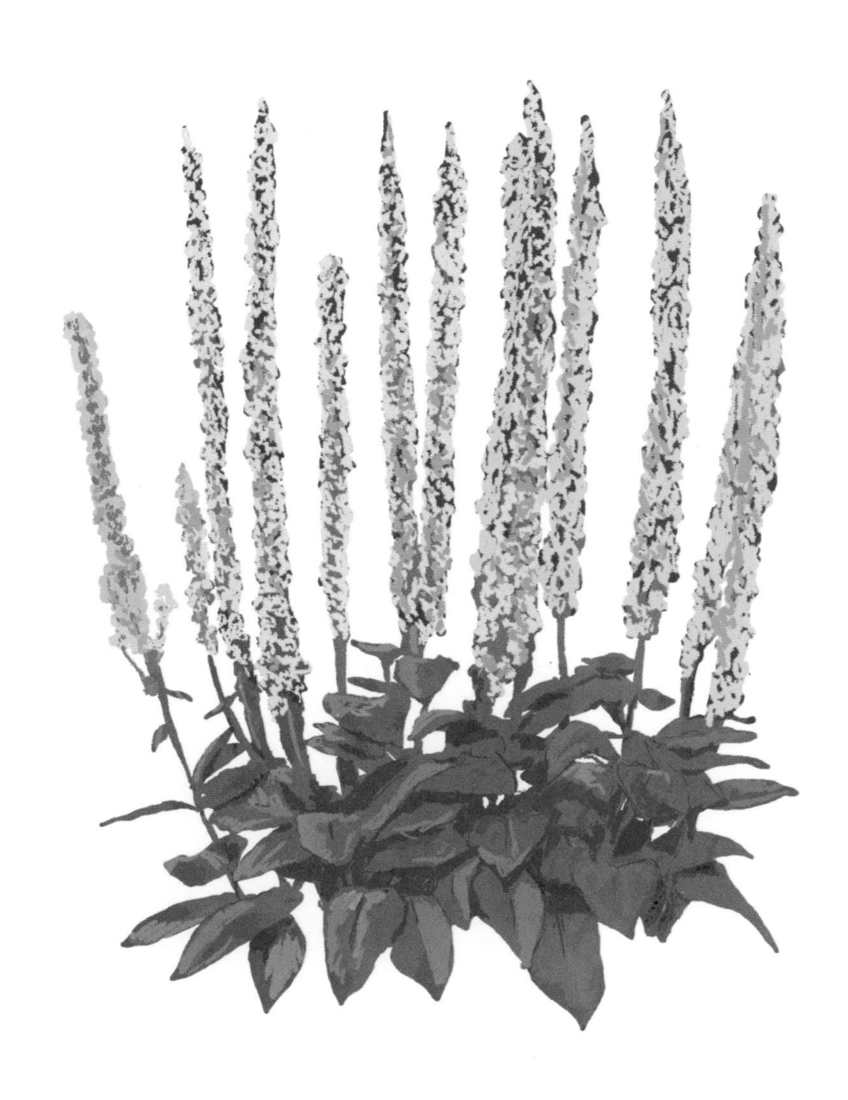

The flower spikes of agrimony grow to about 60cm (2ft) tall.

Agrimony
Agrimonia eupatoria

During Anglo-Saxon times, agrimony was used externally as a wound-healing agent. This use was practised by the French during the fifteenth century, when they applied the herb to soldiers suffering gunshot injuries.

Origins & Characteristics
The agents responsible for the medicinal actions displayed by agrimony have been identified as astringents. These substances have the ability to close wounds and control the flow of blood.

Other medicinal functions of this plant rely on the bitter principles present in the extracts. Bitters can cause the gallbladder to contract and release its stored bile as well as stimulate the flow of digestive juices.

Agrimony can reduce the inflammation of the stomach lining that often results from food allergies. Used externally, this herb can also help to relieve the symptoms of eczema.

Parts Used
Whole plant

Dosage
As a liquid tincture, take 20 drops twice daily before eating. For external application, use as a compress for eczema.

Potential Benefits
- Controls bleeding wounds when applied as a compress
- Assists liver function and digestion
- Helps in some cases of food allergy
- Helps reduce skin irritations from eczema

Cosmetic Uses
The leaves can be used in a facial wash to improve the skin's complexion.

Agrimony flowers open gradually from the bottom of the stem upwards.

Lady's Mantle
Alchemilla vulgaris

The leaves of lady's mantle were considered to hold special magical powers once, so much so that the translation of its botanical name, *Alchemilla*, means 'little magical one'. It has been used for many feminine problems and was thought to restore a lady's beauty, hence its common name.

Origins & Characteristics
In the treatment of menopausal disorders, the astringent and anti-inflammatory properties of lady's mantle help to control irregular bleeding, an effect that prompted its use for menstrual problems in younger women. Taken internally, lady's mantle can help regulate excessive or irregular menstrual bleeding and it can also be used as a treatment for diarrhoea.

Applied externally, its healing properties make it a very useful herb for the treatment of vaginal discharge.

Parts Used
Whole plant

Dosage
As a liquid tincture, take 20 drops twice daily. As a douche, infuse 1 tablespoon dried powder, strain and apply in the morning and evening.

Potential Benefits
- Controls excessive bleeding
- Regulates menstrual bleeding
- Aids in vaginal infections
- Relieves diarrhoea

Cosmetic Uses
The leaves can be used in a lotion as an astringent to help oily skin.

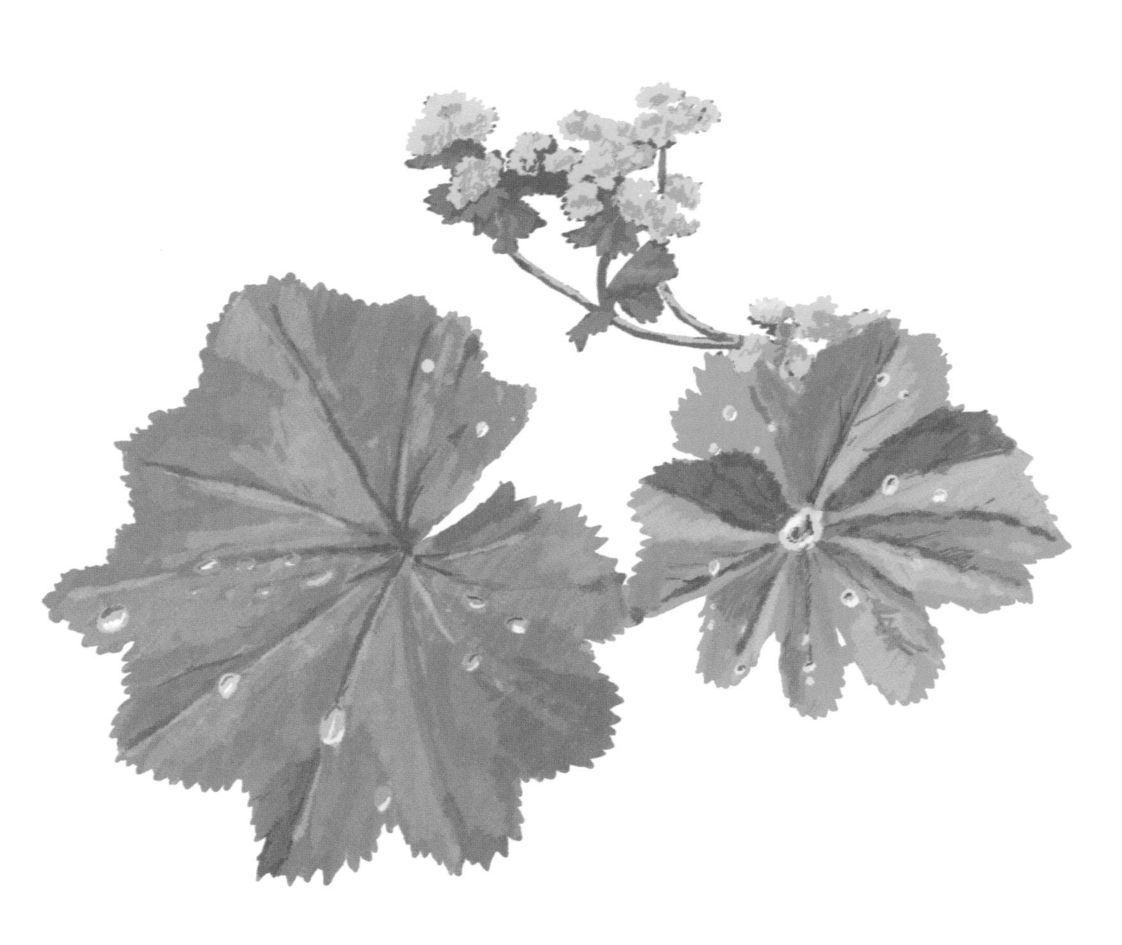

Lady's mantle has slightly hairy leaves, which hold rain and dew in droplets.

Garlic
Allium sativum

It seems that not a day passes without some new benefit of garlic being discovered. The ancient Egyptians actually worshipped the herb and fed it to their slaves to keep them fit and well. Taken internally, garlic's volatile oils keep the lungs clear of infections. The treatment of pneumonia, bronchitis and asthma should be followed up by a preventive dose of garlic daily.

Origins & Characteristics

The risk of heart disease due to cholesterol deposits can be reduced by regular doses of garlic. It has been shown that the 'bad' cholesterol (low-density lipoproteins (LDL)) is reduced, while the 'good' cholesterol (high-density lipoprotein (HDL)) is increased after garlic is ingested. At the same time the stickiness of the blood's platelets (small fragments that cause a clot to form) is dramatically reduced.

Garlic has a powerful antimicrobial action and can be applied directly to infected areas. Fungal infections, often difficult to control, can be reduced by a garlic application. New research is suggesting that garlic contains anticancer substances, but this is still a new area of study.

The aromatic oils contained in garlic give it many of its health-promoting actions. Whenever possible, deodorised garlic preparations should not be used.

Parts Used

Bulb

Dosage

Take 2 or 3 garlic capsules daily with a meal or – as a liquid tincture – take 1 or 2 teaspoons daily.

For external application, crush individual cloves of garlic and apply a paste topically to the affected area.

Potential Benefits

- Protects against heart disease
- Lowers LDL cholesterol
- Can reduce blood pressure
- Exhibits antimicrobial activity
- Kills fungi
- Clears chest infections
- May have cancer-protective action
- Protects against blood clots

Culinary Uses

Garlic enhances the flavours of most foods. Whole, roasted garlic bulbs are sweet and mild. The classic French dressing *aioli* is made out of puréed garlic using 6–12 garlic cloves and a pinch of salt. It originated in Provence, where it is called *beurre de Provence*.

Caution
When applying topically as a paste, do not tape the treatment in place because the oils from the garlic can cause skin burns with chronic exposure.

Eating more than five cloves of garlic at a sitting may cause a stomach upset.

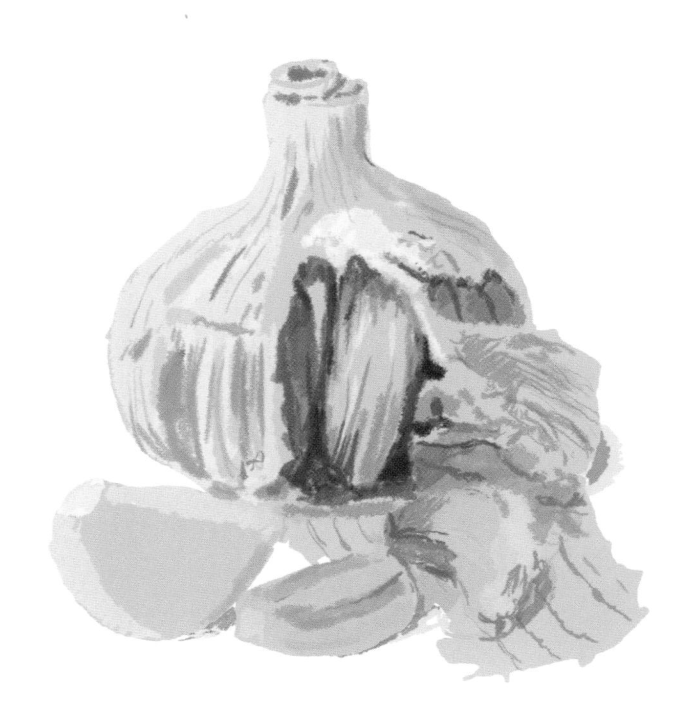

A garlic-rich diet is thought to be very good for your heart.

Chives
Allium schoenoprasum

A member of the lily family first discovered more than 5,000 years ago in China, this common herb can now be found in every food shop. Chives are high in vitamin C and iron. For this reason they are considered to be a highly nutritious food and excellent for building up the blood. Chives also have a mild stimulant effect on the appetite and can aid digestion.

Parts Used
Leaves

Dosage
Eat a large sprig of the whole herb daily.

Potential Benefits
- Restores blood iron levels and combats anemia
- Stimulates appetite
- Aids digestion

Culinary Uses
Used in salads, soups and omelettes, where onions would be too strong, and also as a garnish and in dressings.

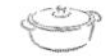 CHIVE AND LEMON VINAIGRETTE

You will need:
- garlic clove
- pinch of salt
- rind of 1 lemon, finely grated
- 4 tbsp lemon juice
- 1½ tsp mustard
- 4 tbsp olive oil
- 2 tsp chives
- black pepper

Put the garlic and a pinch of salt in a bowl and crush together. Add the finely grated lemon rind, lemon juice and mustard and stir until smooth. Slowly pour in the olive oil, whisking constantly until well emulsified. Add the chives and season with pepper. This is delicious spooned over potatoes.

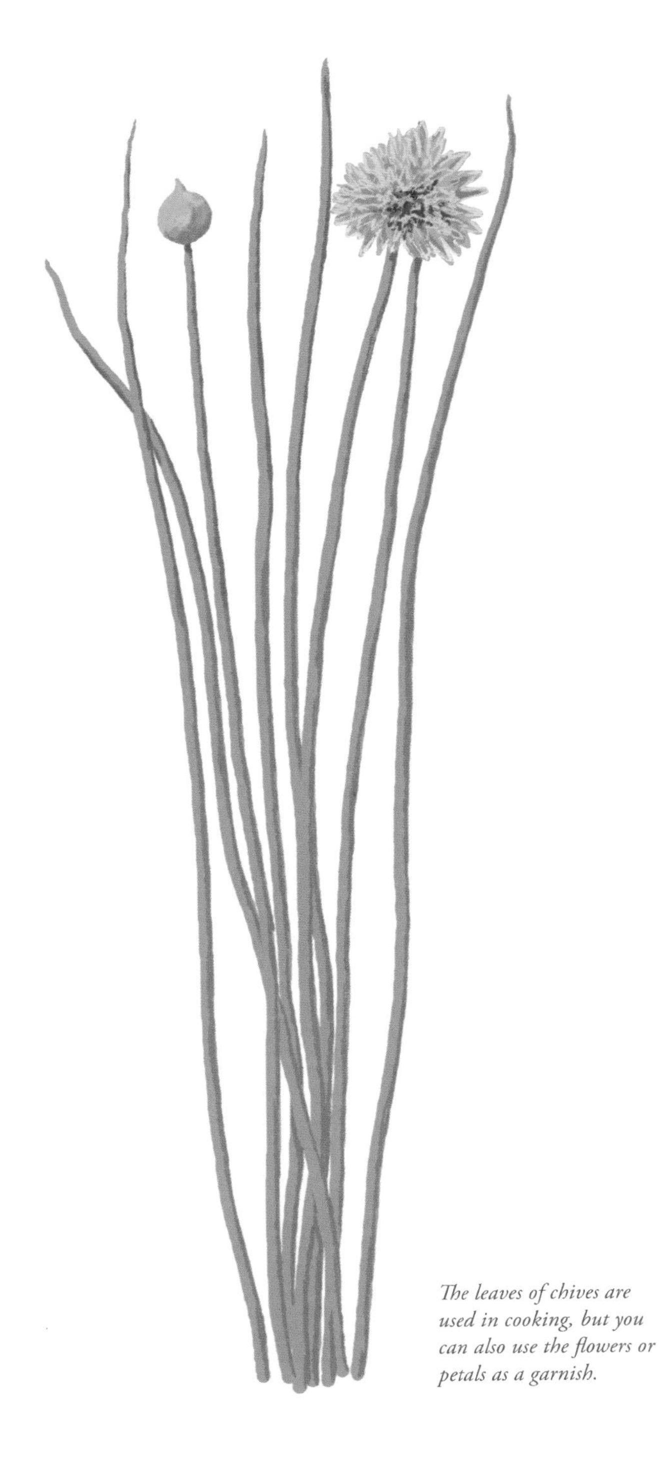

The leaves of chives are used in cooking, but you can also use the flowers or petals as a garnish.

Aloe Vera
Alo barbadensis

Aloe vera is an ancient remedy – it is said that the body of Jesus was wrapped in linen impregnated with aloe vera and myrrh. The juice can be either commercially prepared or extracted from the leaves by scraping it out with the blunt side of a knife.

Origins & Characteristics
Contained within the aloe vera leaf is a special gel that is used in cosmetics as a natural skin moisturiser. A topical application of the juice can help with minor skin burns, sunburn, insect bites and sometimes with eczema.

The juice is taken internally for digestive disorders and inflammation of the stomach. Other benefits have been attributed to aloe vera, such as its ability to act as a natural laxative as well as an appetite stimulant.

Parts Used
Leaves that contain the sap

Dosage
Take 1 tablespoon of the juice twice daily.

For external application, use aloe vera as a cream or lotion on the skin as required.

Potential Benefits
- Keeps skin supple
- Helps speed wound healing
- Reduces inflammation of the stomach
- Acts as a laxative
- Heals sunburn

Cosmetic Uses
Can be made into lotions and creams for soothing irritated and inflamed skin.

Caution
Internal use is not advised during pregnancy. Always seek medical attention for serious burns.

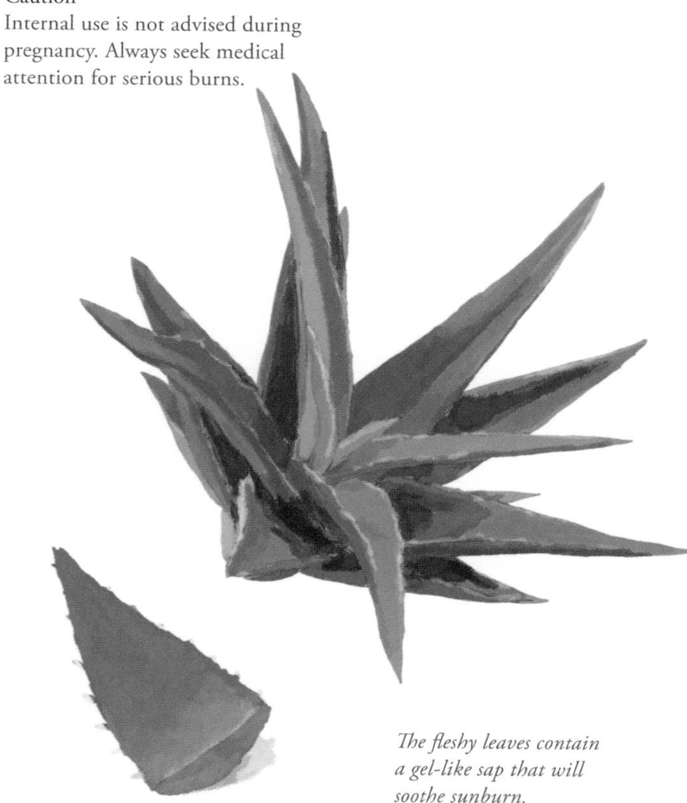

The fleshy leaves contain a gel-like sap that will soothe sunburn.

Marshmallow
Althaea officinalis

Used by the ancient Greeks, marshmallow has long been a favourite herb for the treatment of colds and chest infections including sore throats and coughs. Conditions of the respiratory tract, such as asthma and bronchitis, have also been reported to respond well to this herb.

Origins & Characteristics

Marshmallow's soothing action can be helpful to inflammations of the stomach and lower intestine, especially in conditions such as colitis. Ulcerations of the stomach are eased with the use of marshmallow, which can make a very effective anti-ulcer remedy when combined with licorice.

The peeled and washed root can be given to children to chew on as a teething aid. Used externally, marshmallow can also help heal boils and abscesses.

Parts Used

Leaves and roots

Dosage

Take 2 or 3 tablets (100mg) of dried extract after meals. For external application, use as a poultice for abscesses and boils.

Potential Benefits

- Soothes stomach inflammation
- Helps heal stomach and skin ulcers
- Soothes colitis
- Helps speed recovery from chest injections
- Helps relieve asthma and bronchitis symptoms
- Acts as a teething aid for children

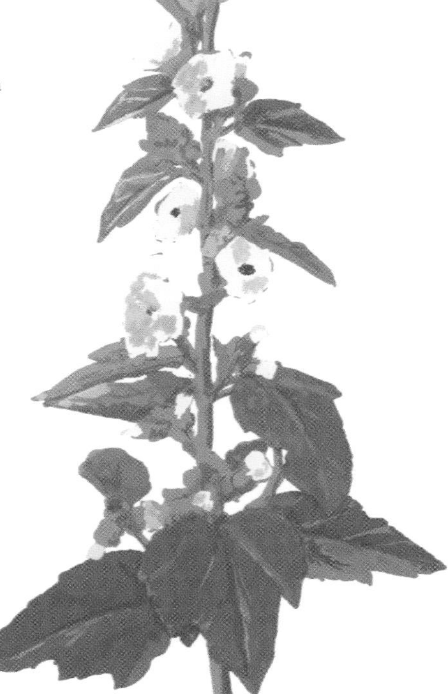

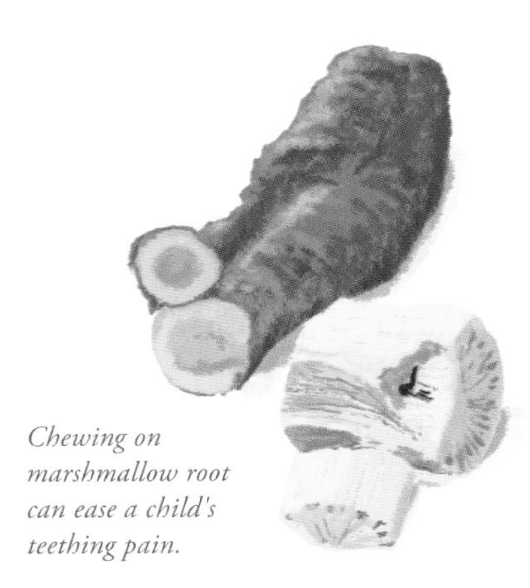

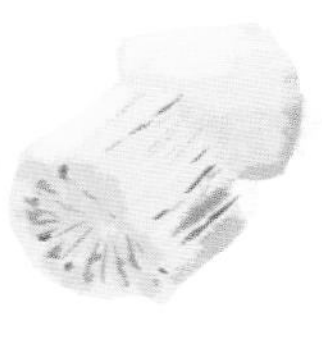

Chewing on marshmallow root can ease a child's teething pain.

Dill
Anethum graveolens

Dill is a popular culinary herb, and it has been used medicinally by doctors since ancient Egyptian and Roman times. The word 'dill' comes from the Saxon word 'dilla', which means to lull or soothe. Taken internally, this herb can relieve an upset stomach and nausea. It has an antispasmodic action that helps to reduce flatulence, stimulate the appetite and aid digestion.

Origins & Characteristics

In babies, dill can be taken to ease colic. The seeds can act as a sedative, and chewing them can sweeten the breath. Dill can also stimulate the flow of breast milk in nursing mothers. Used externally, dill is useful for soothing muscular tension. It can also strengthen fingernails.

Parts Used

Leaves and seeds

Dosage

As dill water, put 2 pinches of dill seeds in 250ml (9fl oz) of water and bring to a boil. As the water changes colour, keep boiling for 1 minute. Strain and cool. Keep it in the fridge.

As a tea, add 2 teaspoons of crushed seeds to 250ml (9fl oz) of boiling water and steep for 5 minutes. To reduce flatulence, drink a cup of the tea before eating.

For external application for muscular tension, use as a compress. For external application to strengthen nails, use as an infusion of dill seeds.

Potential Benefits

- Relieves nausea
- Aids digestion
- Helps reduce colic
- Stimulates the flow of breast milk in nursing mothers
- Soothes muscular tension
- Strengthens fingernails

Culinary Uses

Dill is a popular flavouring in many dishes. Fresh leaves can be used in salads, poultry and fish dishes. Dill pickles are also popular.

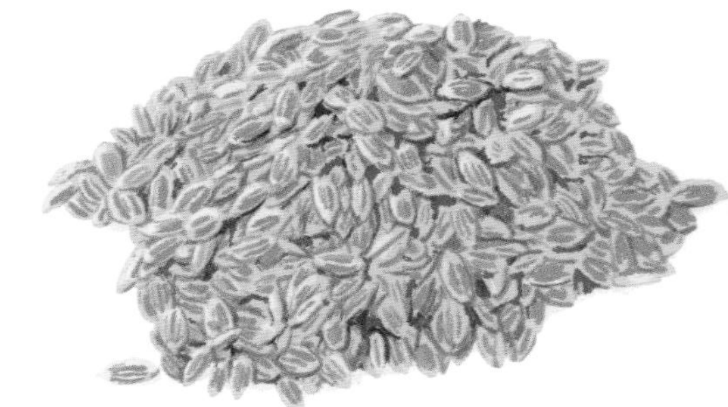

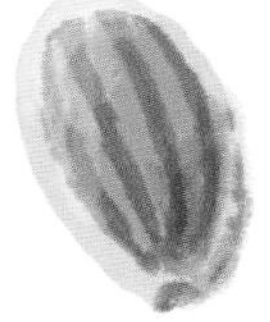

Dill seeds can be crushed and used to make a tea to aid digestion.

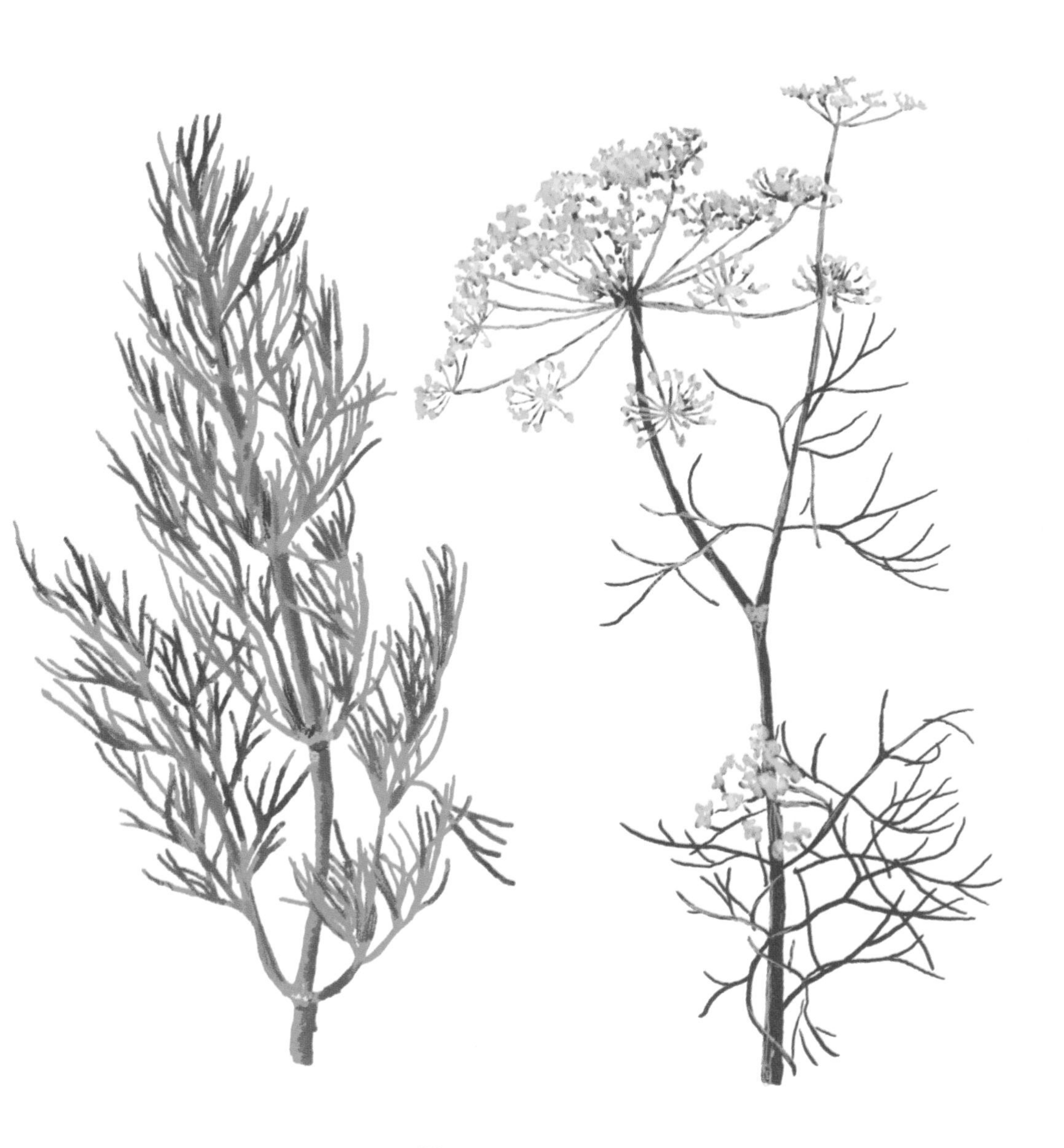

Dill leaves are a common flavouring in fish dishes; try adding the flowers to pickling vinegar.

Angelica
Angelica archangelica

Legend says that angelica was a cure for plague, which has secured it a place in traditional herbal medicine as a protector against evil. Angelica appears to have a beneficial effect on the circulation of blood and body fluids and is a soothing treatment for stomach upsets.

Origins & Characteristics

As a remedy for stomach upsets, gastric ulcers and migraines, angelica can be combined with Roman chamomile (*Anthemis nobilis*). For an effective remedy against bronchitis and congestion of the lungs, angelica can be combined with yarrow (*Achillea millefolium*). An infusion can act as an expectorant in cases of colds and flu.

For the treatment of menstrual cramps and fluid retention, there can be no better herb to take than angelica. The medicinal effect that angelica exerts on the body has offered those suffering from rheumatism and arthritis a noticeable easing of symptoms. This effect may be a result of the removal of inflammatory chemicals accumulated in the tissues. Angelica is also useful in relieving symptoms of cystitis.

Parts Used

Leaves, seeds, stems and roots

Dosage

As a liquid tincture, take 20 drops two or three times a day or 200mg of dried herb daily.

As an infusion, or tea, add 1 tablespoon of dried herb to 500ml (18fl oz) of boiling water.

Potential Benefits

- Eases symptoms of rheumatism and arthritis
- Soothes an upset stomach
- Acts as an antispasmodic to soothe menstrual cramps
- Relieves symptoms of cystitis
- Acts as an expectorant for chest infections

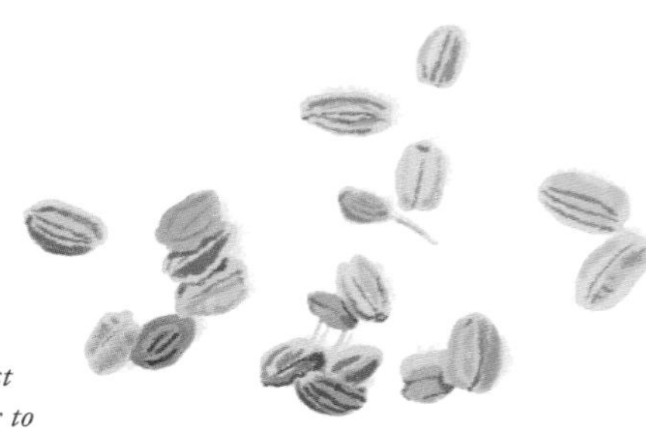

Angelica seeds are most often used in sweets or to flavour liqueurs.

Culinary Uses

Angelica leaves will give a salad a lively and aromatic flavour. The best-known application for angelica is its candied form, used for cake decoration. This is not difficult to make at home. After collecting angelica stems, place them in boiling water until they are tender enough to remove the outer skins. Return the peeled stems to the pan and bring to a boil again. Cool the stems and add an equal weight of sugar to the stems, cover and leave for two days. Then place the stems and the syrup in a pan and bring to a boil again. Preheat an oven to 100°C (200°F) and place the stems (after sprinkling with icing sugar) on a tray until they have completely dried out. Store in an airtight jar.

Caution

Avoid during pregnancy as large doses of angelica may disrupt blood pressure. This herb should also be avoided by people who suffer from high blood pressure. Some people suffer sunlight sensitivity due to a substance called furocoumarin present in the plant, which may also cause skin irritation.

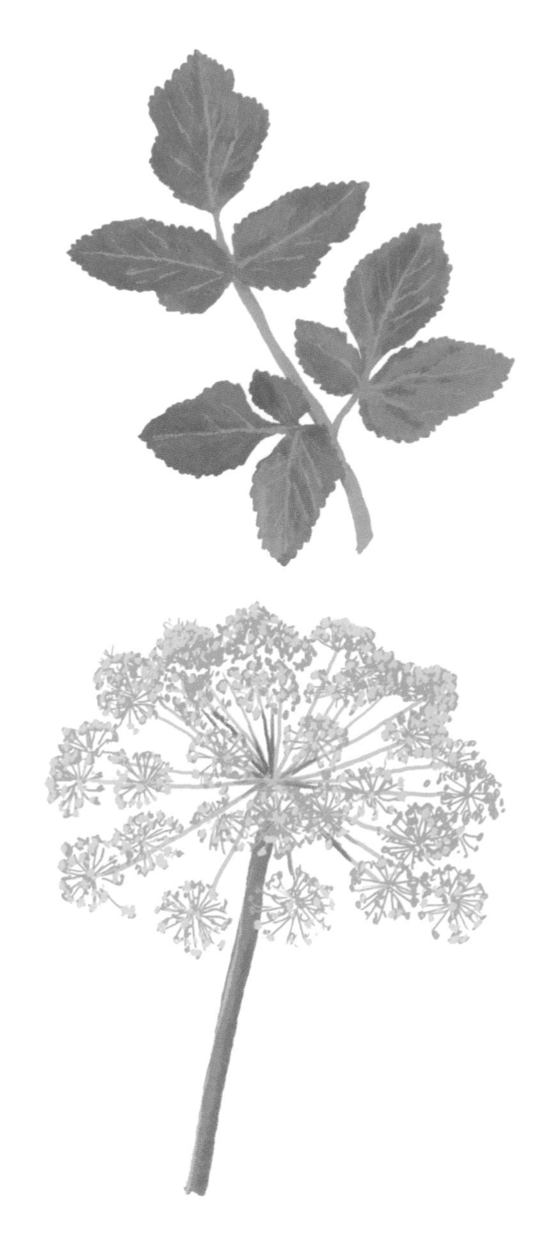

Angelica grows to 2m (6ft) or more. Its leaves, flowers, stems, seeds and roots are all used.

Roman Chamomile
Anthemis nobilis

The ancient Egyptians make reference to the use of chamomile in their writings, making it another herb with a long and trusted history. Chamomile has been taken for centuries to calm the nerves and induce rest. When taken internally, the herb assists in soothing an upset stomach and menstrual cramps and dulling muscular aches and travel sickness, as chamomile has an excellent antispasmodic action.

Origins & Characteristics

Chamomile tea can be drunk to help reduce nasal congestion and lower temperatures associated with colds and flu. A tincture is especially useful for childhood teething problems, as chamomile has natural painkilling properties. It is also safe to use for children.

Chamomile is an excellent antiseptic and can help to relieve urinary infections, including cystitis. The best treatment method is to drink copious amounts of chamomile tea, sit in a chamomile bath and place hot compresses on the lower abdomen.

Chamomile is also a mild diuretic, which helps reduce fluid retention. This may be helpful in premenstrual syndrome as it may alleviate bloating. This herb is a good anti-depressant and may relieve anxiety and tension. An aromatherapy application may be beneficial for helping depression.

An external application rapidly soothes sunburn, haemorrhoids, skin wounds, mastitis and skin ulcers. An immune-stimulating action has also been reported.

Parts Used

Flowers and essential oil

Dosage

As a tincture, take 15–20 drops twice daily. As a tea, follow the manufacturer's instructions.

As an aromatherapy application, use 6 drops of essential oil mixed together with 2 teaspoons of almond oil. Massage in the usual way.

For external application, use as a cream or compress.

Potential Benefits

- Calms the nerves
- Reduces internal inflammation, especially of the stomach
- Reduces flatulence
- Aids in teething pain
- Helps reduce nasal congestion
- Soothes irritated skin and skin wounds
- Eases menstrual cramps

Cosmetic Uses
Chamomile can be used in a cleansing milk for dry and chapped skin and in a shampoo for fair hair. It is also useful as a hand cream. A few drops of chamomile oil can be added for a relaxing bath.

Caution
Avoid using the essential oil during early pregnancy as it can stimulate menstruation.

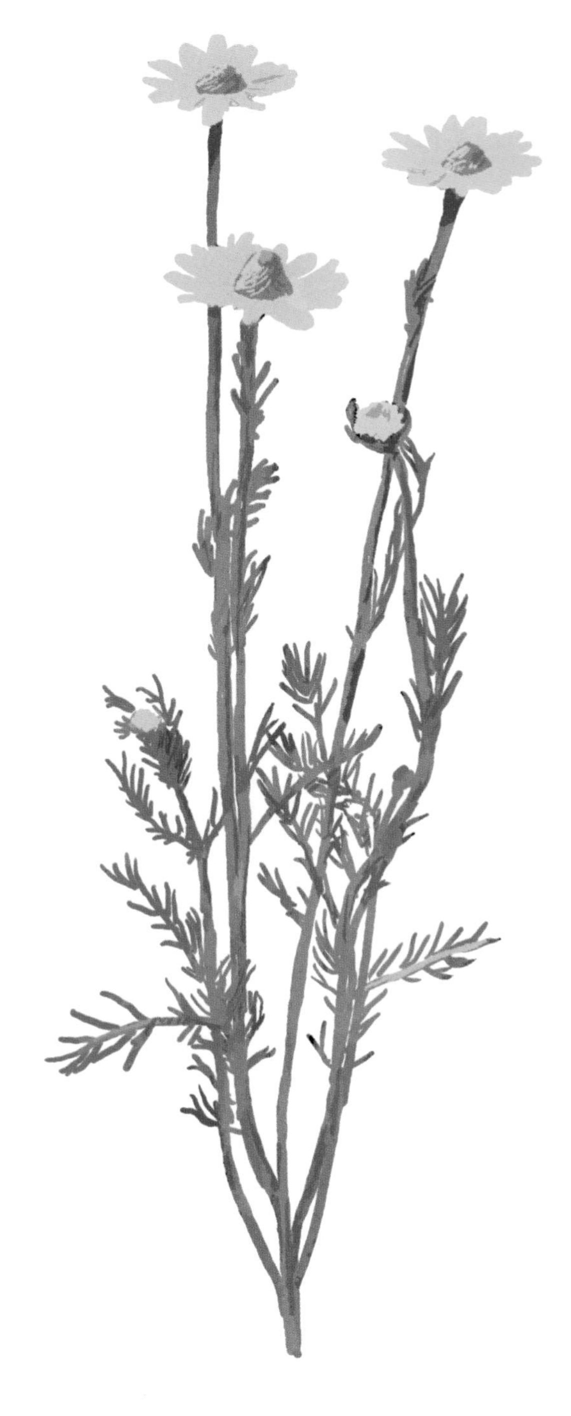

Chamomile is one of the most ancient healing herbs, best known as a tea.

Celery
Apium graveolens

Celery was present in the tomb of Tutankhamun (c.1370–1352 B.C.) and has been used as a food and spice for as long as records have been kept. Celery can reduce blood pressure, probably as a result of its diuretic action. Inflammation of the bladder, gout and arthritis all show improvements when treated with celery extracts. An external application helps in cases of fungal infections, and drinking celery juice has been reported to stimulate menstruation. For this reason its use is not advised during pregnancy.

Parts Used
Whole plant

Dosage
Drink a small tumbler or 150ml (5fl oz) of fresh juice daily (best diluted 50:50 with water). Or add 5 drops of oil extract to a tumbler or 150ml (5fl oz) of water daily.

For external application, add 6 drops of essential oil to 2 teaspoons almond oil and massage into the affected area twice a day to eradicate fungal infections.

Potential Benefits
- Acts as a diuretic
- Has anti-inflammatory properties
- Promotes menstruation
- Reduces arthritis symptoms

Culinary Uses
Celery can be washed and eaten raw or added to casseroles.

Caution
Avoid concentrated extracts or tinctures during pregnancy.

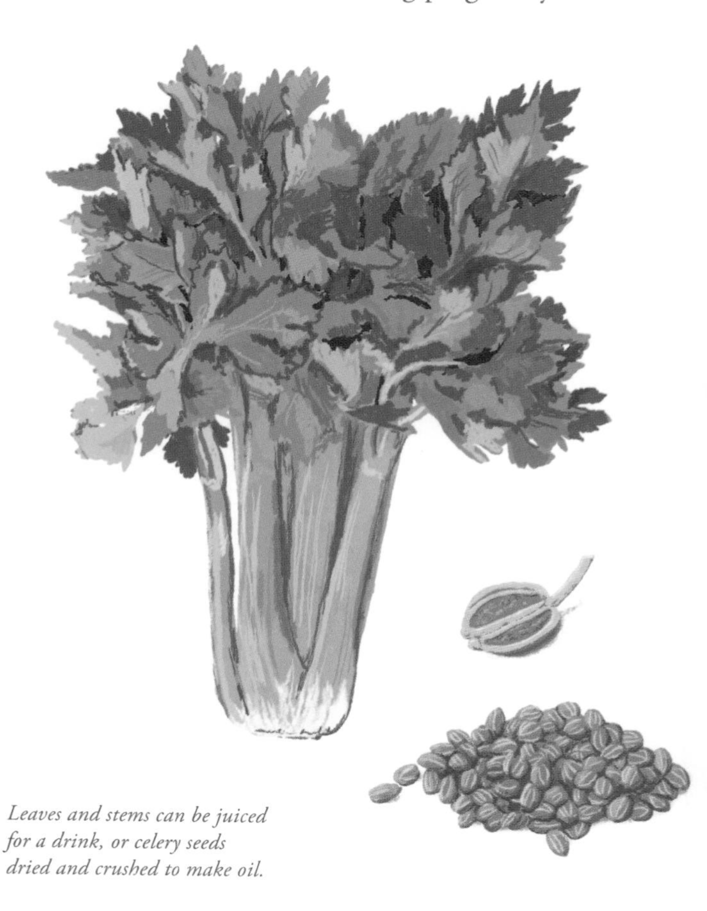

Leaves and stems can be juiced for a drink, or celery seeds dried and crushed to make oil.

Burdock
Arctium lappa

Burdock has sweet roots and bitter leaves. The roots contain a mucilaginous substance that has a calming and anti-inflammatory action on the stomach. In herbal medicine burdock has traditionally been used internally for the treatment of psoriasis, eczema, rheumatism and gout. In Chinese medicine, burdock was said to be of benefit in treating pneumonia and throat infections. Burdock also acts as a mild diuretic and detoxifying agent in chronic diseases, such as arthritis.

Parts Used
Leaves and roots

Dosage
Take 2 or 3 tablets (100mg) of dried extract after meals.

For external application, use as a poultice for abscesses and boils.

Potential Benefits
- Soothes stomach inflammation
- Helps heal stomach and skin ulcers
- Soothes colitis
- Helps speed recovery from chest injections
- Helps relieve asthma and bronchitis symptoms
- Acts as a teething aid for children

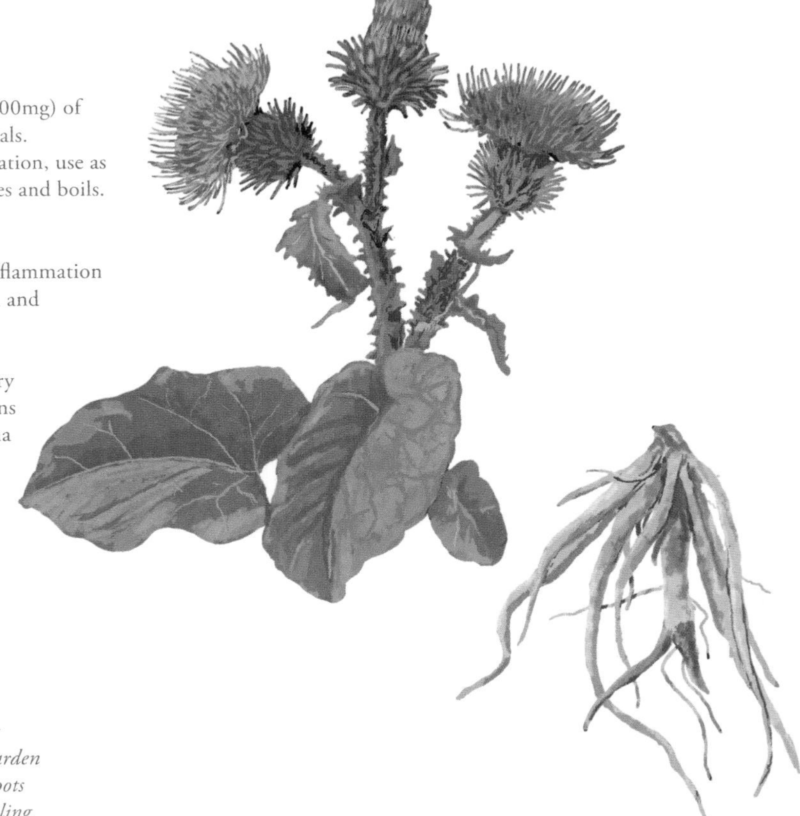

Burdock flowers bring autumn colour to a garden or roadside, but the roots are most useful in healing.

Uva-ursi (Bearberry; or Upland Cranberry)

Arctostaphylos uva-ursi

This plant has several common names, and is also known as bearberry or the upland cranberry. It is a small shrub that has been used to treat urinary tract infections for centuries, but it also has many other potential health benefits.

Origins & Characteristics

The bacterium *E. coli* is very susceptible to the chemicals found in uva-ursi and the antibacterial agent arbutin has given this herb a special place in the treatment of urinary tract infections, especially cystitis.

In addition to its antibiotic activity, uva-ursi has a beneficial diuretic action that helps in the elimination of the infective agent. Uva-ursi also has high astringent actions that can help relieve minor vaginal infections.

Parts Used

Leaves

Dosage

Take 2 tablets (100mg) of dried herb daily until your symptoms are relieved.

For use as a douche, infuse 1 tablespoon of dried herb, strain and apply.

Potential Benefits

- Soothes symptoms of bladder and mild kidney infections
- Acts as a diuretic
- Relieves minor vaginal infections
- Reduces symptoms of cystitis

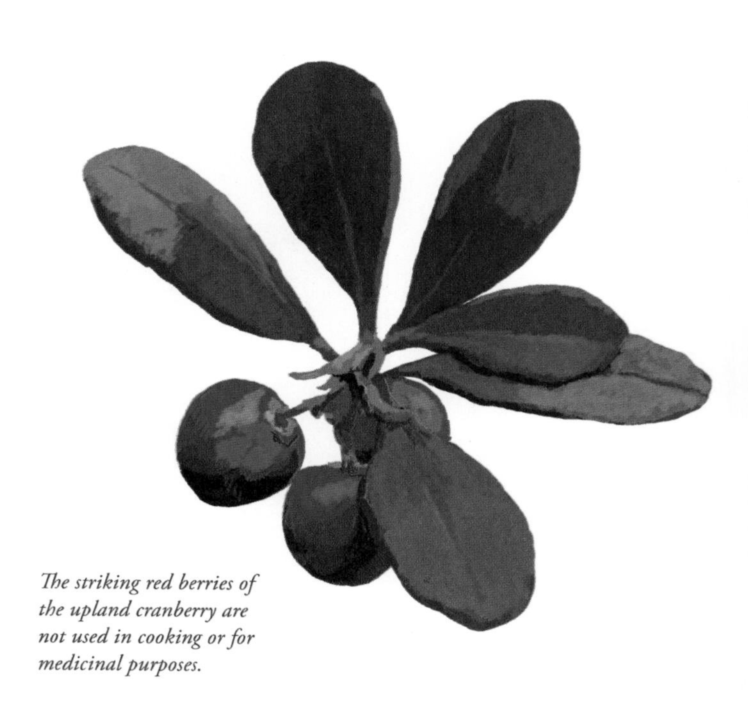

The striking red berries of the upland cranberry are not used in cooking or for medicinal purposes.

Horseradish
Armoracia rusticana

This very aromatic herb contains oils that can control microbial infections. A horseradish poultice has been traditionally used over areas of infection, especially over the chest for the treatment of pleurisy. The drawing properties of horseradish are said to clear the infection.

Origins & Characteristics
Horseradish is an excellent remedy for lung infections. During the elimination of the oils from the lung, the antibacterial activity of the herb permeates through the entire lung, cleansing as it goes. Horseradish can even help to lower a fever by increasing perspiration as the volatile oils are eliminated.

As a diuretic, horseradish is quite effective, but its stimulating action on digestion is greater.

Parts Used
Leaves and roots

Dosage
For external application, use as a poultice. Add the shredded herb to a mixture of flour and water to make a paste. Apply to the affected area and cover.

As a liquid tincture, take 20 drops twice daily after eating.

Mix the shredded herb with honey and hot water for an effective cold remedy.

Potential Benefits
- Acts as a mild diuretic
- Cleanses the lungs
- Acts as an antimicrobial agent
- Clears infections
- Stimulates digestion

Culinary Uses
Try the fresh leaves in salads or with smoked fish. Roast beef would not be the same without a serving of horseradish sauce.

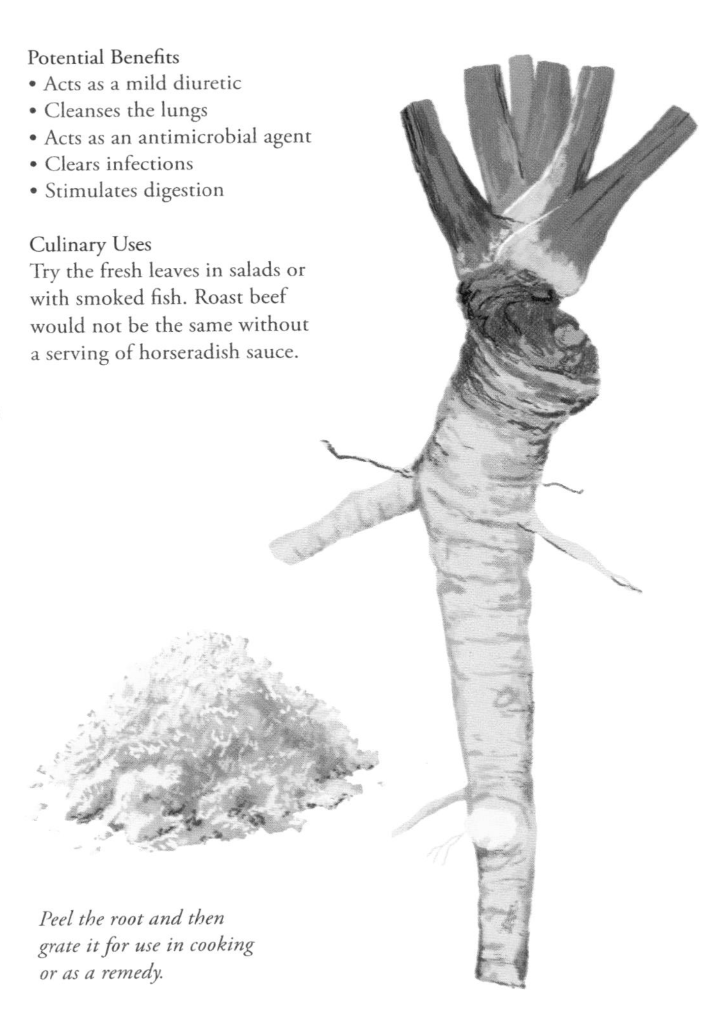

Peel the root and then grate it for use in cooking or as a remedy.

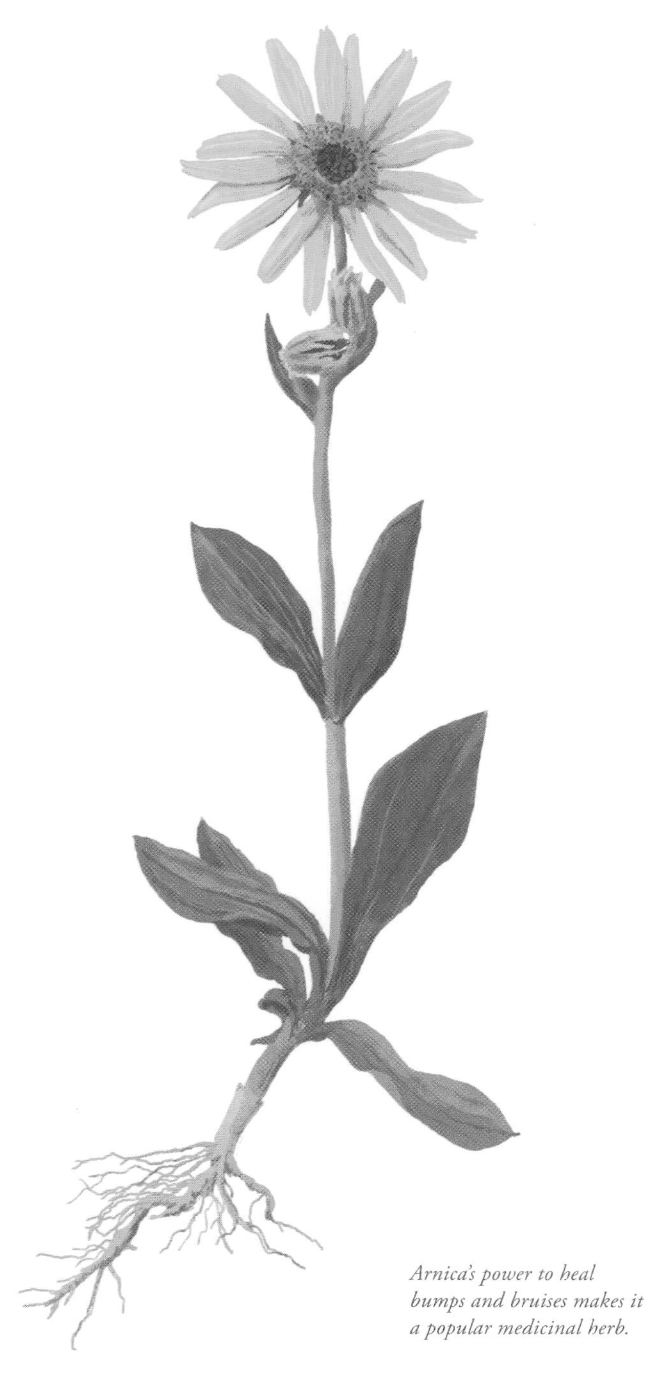

Arnica's power to heal bumps and bruises makes it a popular medicinal herb.

Arnica
Arnica montana

Arnica rose to fame during the eighteenth century as a cure-all. Although many claims were exaggerated, arnica still holds a special place in herbal medicine today. Recent studies have suggested that internal use should be avoided, but some homeopathic remedies do use small internal doses to treat ailments. Always consult a medical practitioner before using arnica to self-treat.

Origins & Characteristics

The arnica plant produces a single, large, yellow flower that lasts throughout the summer. The leaves are picked during the growing season.

Its external use is widespread. When used on the skin, arnica has remarkable properties and can assist the healing process. Bruises, cuts and abrasions all respond very well to arnica cream.

Sports injuries, when caught early, improve quickly with an arnica preparation and arnica liniments are available for the treatment of muscular rheumatism and arthritis.

Parts Used

Leaves

Dosage

Internal use of this herb should be undertaken with professional guidance only, but over-the-counter homeopathic preparations containing arnica are considered to be very safe.

Try using a 4x or 6x strength tincture remedy at a dose of 5–10 drops taken three times a day about a half hour before eating. Take this remedy with water only.

For external application, follow the manufacturer's instructions.

Potential Benefits

- Reduces inflammation in tissues
- Stimulates the healing process
- Reduces muscular spasm and joint inflammation
- Soothes irritated skin

Cosmetic Uses

Can be made into creams to stimulate the skin's circulation.

Caution

Do not take internally unless under professional advice as an overdose can prove fatal. Avoid during pregnancy.

External use may cause skin irritation. Never apply arnica to broken skin.

Southernwood
Artemisia abrotanum

Southernwood's use dates back to ancient China, where it was used externally for the treatment of inflamed or burned skin. The herb is very bitter, and its effectiveness can be ascribed to the high concentrations of astringents present in the plant extracts.

Origins & Characteristics
This plant has a tonic effect on the digestive system, stimulating an improved bile and digestive juice flow. The muscles of the uterus can react strongly to this botanical substance, and menstruation can be induced by taking the extract, so it must never be taken during pregnancy.

This herb has also been reported to help in expelling intestinal worms in children.

Parts Used
Leaves

Dosage
As a liquid tincture, take 20 drops daily. For external application, use as a compress for irritated skin.

Potential Benefits
- Stimulates digestion
- Aids in the flow of bile and, therefore, the digestion of fat
- Helps in painful menstruation
- Soothes irritated skin
- Helps expel worms in children

Caution
Avoid during pregnancy.

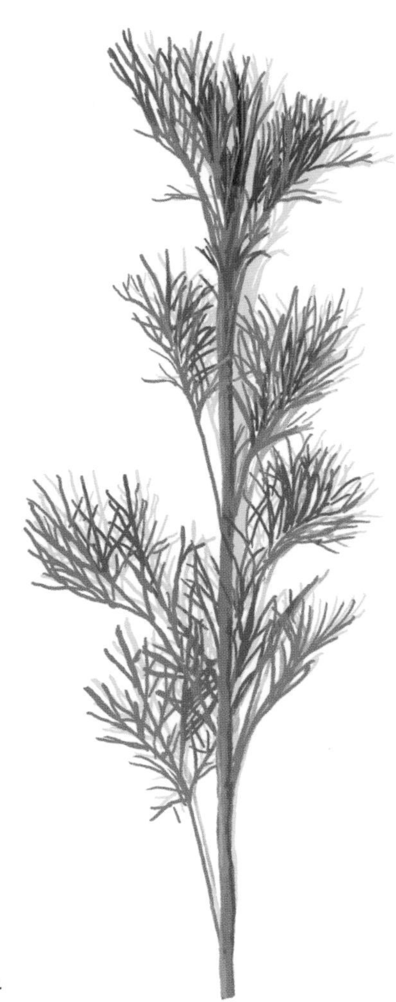

Southernwood's feathery foliage can be used as a compress on irritated skin.

Astragalus

Astragalus membranaceus

Astragalus was held in high esteem by the ancient Chinese, who incorporated it into many of their medicinal formulas. The herb has a sweet taste and has been used in traditional medicine to help to stimulate the immune system, lungs, liver and spleen.

Origins & Characteristics

Astragalus also stimulates the circulatory system and acts as a heart tonic. Beneficial effects of lowering high blood pressure and blood glucose levels have also been reported.

Herbal practitioners may suggest using this herb during treatment with chemotherapy as it stimulates the immune system, but this approach needs cooperation between the herbalist and doctor and should not be taken without supervision.

Parts Used

Root

Dosage

As a liquid tincture, take 15–20 drops daily.

Potential Benefits

- Has a general tonic effect
- May help lower blood glucose levels
- Stimulates the immune system
- Aids the flow of bile and liver function
- May help lower blood pressure

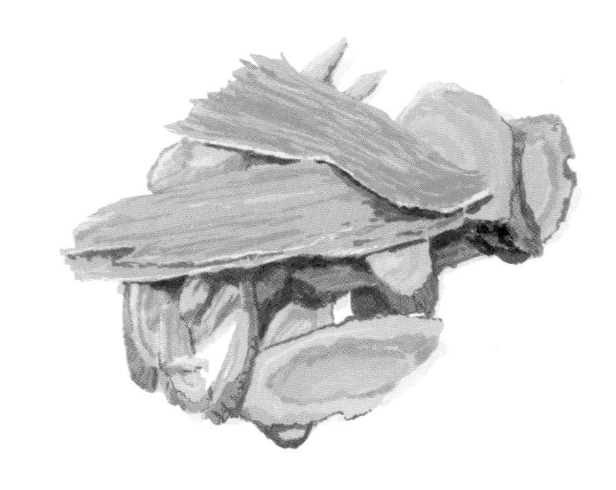

Astragalus root is dried and cut into slices or lengthwise slivers.

Oats
Avena sativa

Oats can be considered a food as well as a herb. Oats are a rich source of vitamins (especially vitamin E), carbohydrates and protein. The heart, nerves and thymus glands all benefit from a dose of oats. The high silica content makes oats a good food to eat if your cholesterol level is high.

Origins & Characteristics
As a remedy for exhaustion, oats act as a nutritive nervine or nerve tonic and may help in cases of depression. For eczema, oats form a good poultice, which helps to reduce inflammation and irritation.

Parts Used
Seeds

Dosage
As a liquid tincture, take 25 drops twice daily.

For external application, use as a poultice. Mix oats into a thick, sticky mass with a little hot water and apply to the skin.

Potential Benefits
- Acts as a heart and nerve tonic
- Lowers cholesterol levels
- May help relieve depression
- Eases symptoms of eczema

Cosmetic Uses
Use oatmeal for facial scrubs to cleanse the skin.

Culinary Uses
Cooked oats are made into porridge. Oats can form the basis for pancakes.

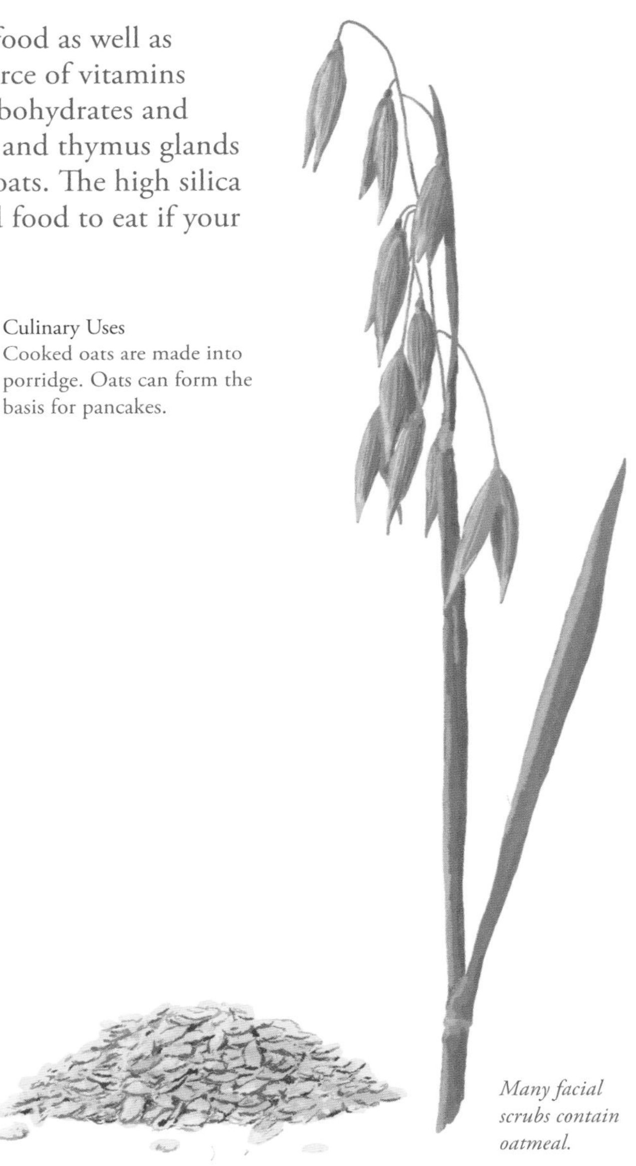

Many facial scrubs contain oatmeal.

Borage
Borago officinalis

A familiar herb to cooks, borage has been associated with mood-enhancing effects. The exact constituents of this plant have not been identified, but its reputation for 'lifting the spirits' dates back to 1597, when John Gerard included it in his book *The Herball*, or *Generall Historie of Plantes*. In this book, borage was said to 'drive away sorrow and increase the joy of the mind'. The leaves and flowers were often made into wines and given to men and women to make them 'glad and merry'.

Origins & Characteristics

Borage has a very high GLA (gamma linoleic acid) content – higher than evening primrose oil – which helps to reduce menstrual cramps. Borage tea is said to be good for lowering high temperatures as it has an excellent diaphoretic action. This makes it an ideal remedy for relieving cold and flu symptoms.

Parts Used

Leaves, flowers, oil and seeds

Dosage

As a liquid tincture, take 15–20 drops twice daily. Borage oil can be taken at a dose of 500mg daily. As a tea, add 2 teaspoons of herbs to 600ml (1 pint) of boiling water and infuse for 5 minutes.

Potential Benefits

- Has mood-lifting effects
- Helps in cases of premenstrual tension
- Helps dermatitis and other skin irritations such as eczema
- Lowers high temperatures

Culinary Uses

Try adding chopped borage to vegetables and pasta dishes, or sprinkle the leaves on salads as a garnish.

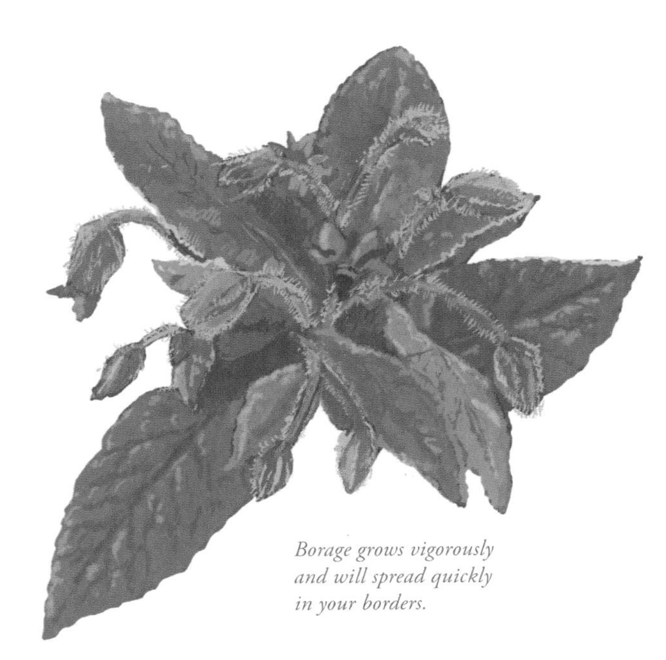

Borage grows vigorously and will spread quickly in your borders.

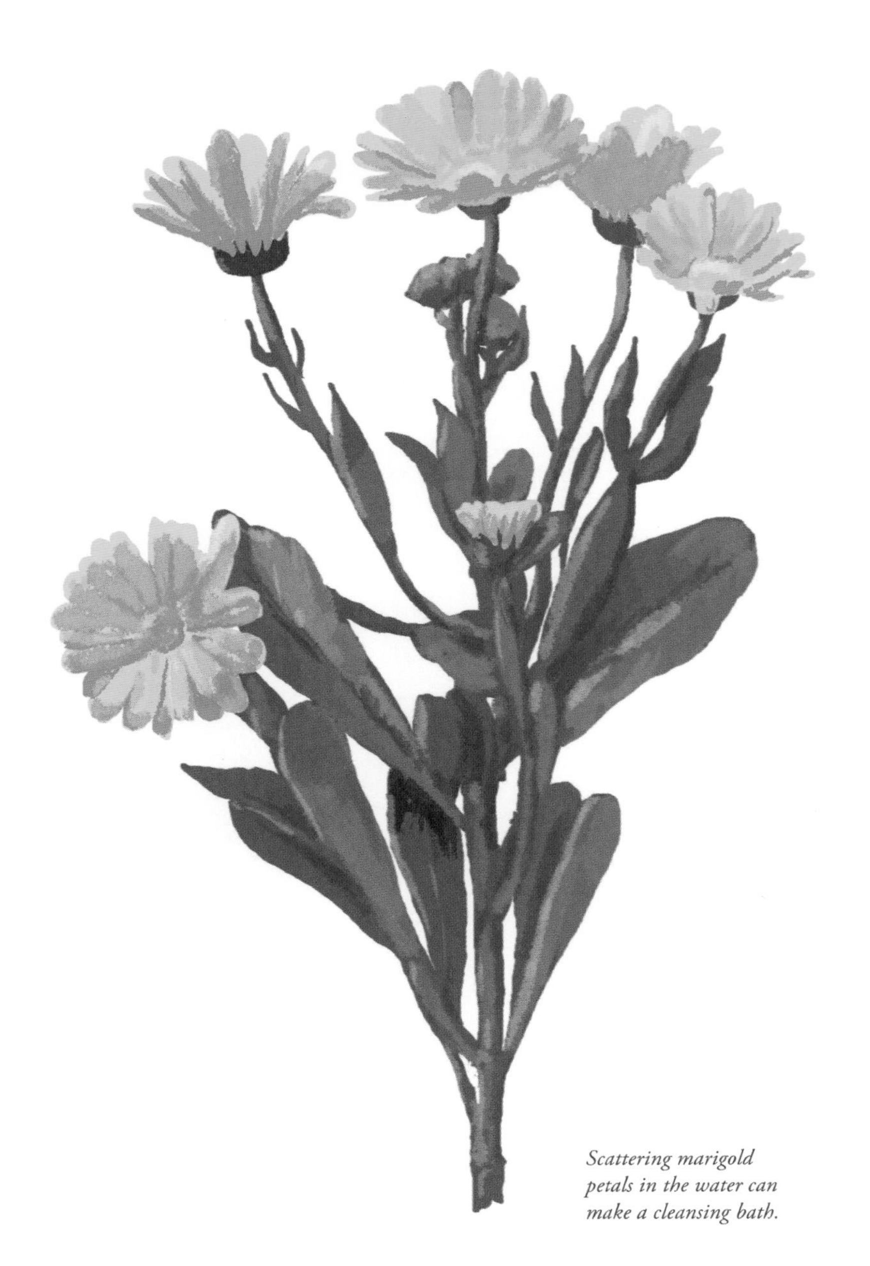

Scattering marigold petals in the water can make a cleansing bath.

Calendula
Calendula officinalis

Also known as marigold, calendula has a long history in herbal medicine. Initially used to dye fabric, as a food and in cosmetics, calendula also contains many oils that have health-promoting properties.

Origins & Characteristics

Used externally, calendula can reduce inflamed skin and sunburn and promote the healing of wounds. It can also be used to relieve cracked nipples when breastfeeding. The oil can reduce earache. Its internal use can help to soothe stomach ulcers and inflammation.

Studies have confirmed the effectiveness of calendula in treating menstrual cramps.

Parts Used

Flower petals

Dosage

As a tea, follow manufacturer's directions. As a liquid tincture, take 15 drops twice daily.

For external application, use as a cream, compress or poultice for wounds and inflamed skin as needed.

Potential Benefits

- Reduces inflammation
- Eases menstrual cramps
- Soothes irritated and damaged skin, such as minor burns
- Relieves earache

Cosmetic Uses

May be used in a cream to help dry and irritated skin and sore or cracked nipples.

The petals can be used in the bath to cleanse and tone the skin.

Cayenne
Capsicum frutescens

Cayenne has been used medicinally (externally as a cream) to treat chronic pain syndromes such as post-shingles neuralgia and osteoarthritis. It also has the ability to stimulate the circulatory system and can be used to treat varicose veins.

Origins & Characteristics

There has been much interest in cayenne since it was shown to reduce sensitivity to pain. Cayenne has the ability to overstimulate nerves and deplete their stores of chemicals that relay information to the brain. In effect, it means that the nerves cannot send pain messages.

Cayenne contains liberal amounts of vitamins, especially the B complex and vitamin C. This herb has beneficial effects on the blood's fat content by reducing the levels of low-density lipoprotein (bad cholesterol) and triglycerides.

This herb is also used to treat asthma and pleurisy, as it stimulates the release of adrenaline that opens up the airways. It should always be taken with caution and always under supervision.

Parts Used

Fruits

Dosage

Take 1 or 2 tablets (100mg) of dried herb with a meal.

For external application, apply cream daily for no longer than one month.

Potential Benefits

- Relieves pain in cases of chronic neuralgia (external use)
- Reduces pain of osteoarthritis
- Stimulates digestion
- Stimulates circulation
- Protects the heart from excessive cholesterol
- May relieve pleurisy
- Eases varicose vein symptoms

Caution

Do not apply cayenne cream to broken skin.

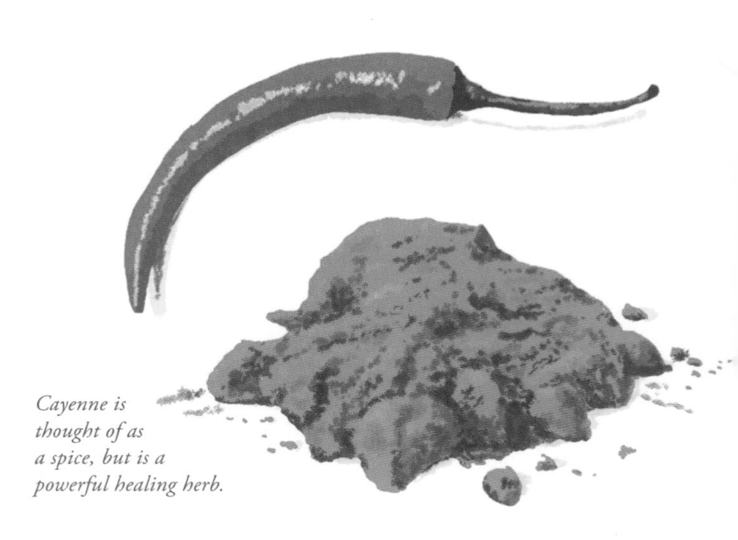

Cayenne is thought of as a spice, but is a powerful healing herb.

Papaya
Carica papaya

This is nature's very best digestive aid. The enzymes contained in papaya break down proteins very efficiently. If you find that you bloat after eating, try some papaya after a meal or as the basis for your dessert, perhaps in a fruit salad.

Origins & Characteristics
As a remedy for intestinal worms (threadworms and roundworms), papaya works in almost all cases. The papain content of papaya can also help to speed wound healing and soften scar tissue.

Parts Used
Leaves, fruits, seeds and sap

Dosage
For a worm remedy, take 2 tablets (50mg) of dried extract daily.

For a digestive aid, take the tablets during every meal or drink fresh juice after each meal.

Potential Benefits
- Aids digestion
- Relieves abdominal bloating after eating
- Helps eliminate worms

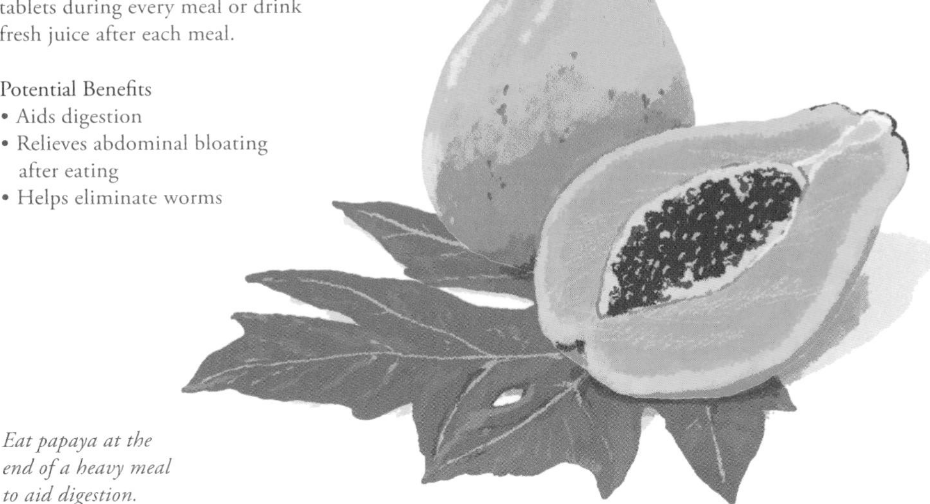

Eat papaya at the end of a heavy meal to aid digestion.

Caraway
Carum carvi

The unmistakable smell of caraway comes from the high concentration of a volatile oil known as carvone, which makes up 40–60 per cent of the oils contained within the seeds. Caraway is well known for reducing colic in babies and flatulence in adults. Its calming effect on the bowels is based on its antispasmodic activity on the bowels' muscular wall.

Origins & Characteristics
Adding some caraway seeds to an herbal tea will help in fighting a cold or flu. Caraway can also be used to stimulate the flow of breast milk in nursing mothers.

Parts Used
Seeds, leaves, roots and oil extract

Dosage
Add a pinch of seeds to an herbal tea. Add 2 or 3 drops of infant colic formula to each feeding to combat colic.

Potential Benefits
- Eases colic in babies
- Reduces flatulence and aids digestion in adults
- Helps fight colds, flu and bronchitis
- Stimulates the flow of breast milk

Culinary Uses
Try adding caraway seeds to cooking water for vegetables. Add to cheese fondues, bread mixes and goulash. It is good when added to lentil dishes.

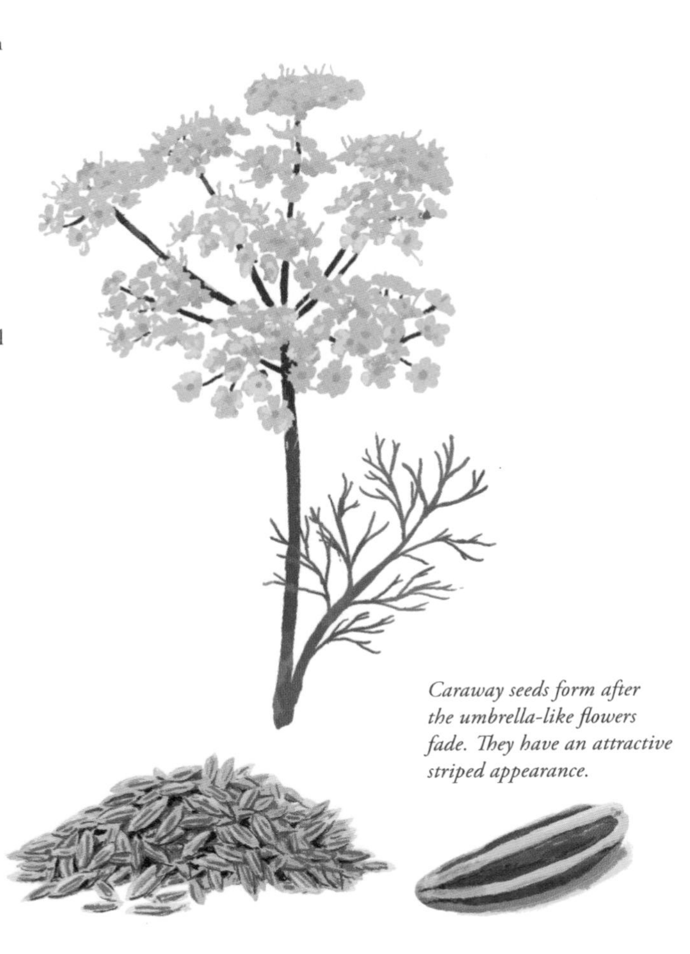

Caraway seeds form after the umbrella-like flowers fade. They have an attractive striped appearance.

Centaury
Centaurium erythraea

Growing in large numbers in very dry and grassy places, centaury is easily spotted by its characteristic spiky appearance. All parts of this bitter-tasting plant are used in herbal medicine, especially the stems. A liquid extract of centaury still tastes bitter even after it is diluted 3,500 times.

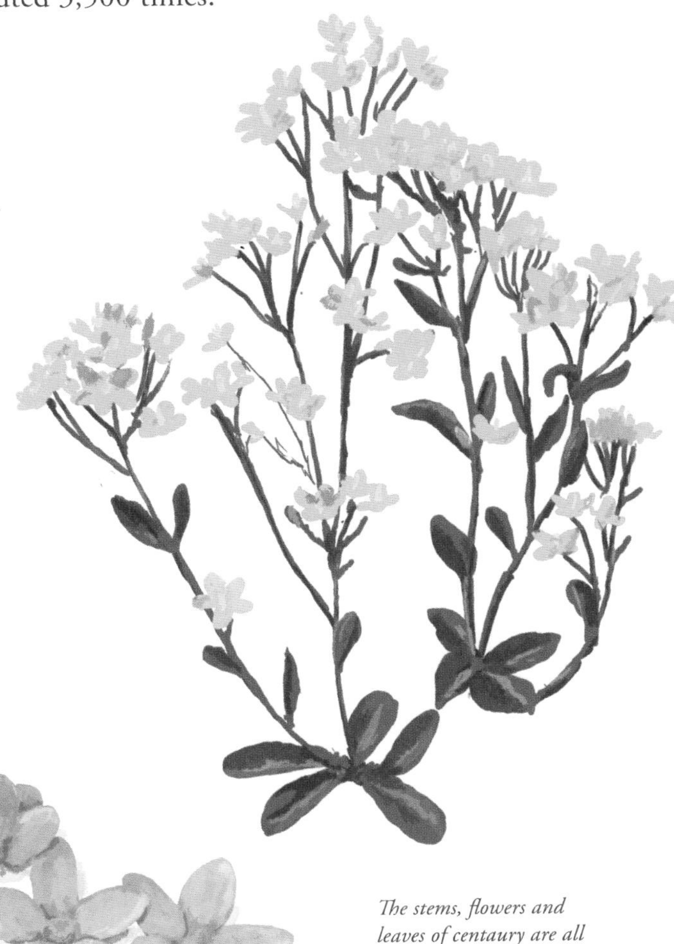

Origins & Characteristics
As a medicine, centaury has general tonic properties, but its most important function is the stimulation of stomach activity and the secretion of gastric juices. It can also be used to relieve dyspepsia, stimulate the appetite and aid in poor digestion. If taken in large doses, it can have a laxative effect.

Parts Used
Whole plant

Dosage
As a liquid tincture, take 25 drops before each meal.

Potential Benefits
- Stimulates appetite
- Aids poor digestion
- Helps reduce stomach gas formation
- Relieves dyspepsia
- Has laxative effects in large doses

The stems, flowers and leaves of centaury are all used in herbal medicine.

Gotu Kola
Centella asiatica

First used by Ayurvedic healers in India, gotu kola has played an important role in controlling the symptoms of stress by inducing a state of relaxation, like a nerve tonic. This herb has been shown to improve immune function and stimulate resistance to infection.

Origins & Characteristics
Similar to ginkgo (*Ginkgo biloba*), gotu kola stimulates the circulatory system, bringing blood to all parts of the body and stabilizing the cells that make up the walls of the blood vessels.

Parts Used
Whole plant

Dosage
Take up to 2 tablets (100mg) of dried extract daily.

Potential Benefits
- Improves resistance to disease
- Induces a state of relaxation
- Relaxes the nervous system
- Stimulates circulation to the entire body

Caution
Avoid during pregnancy. Do not use if you have an overactive thyroid gland.

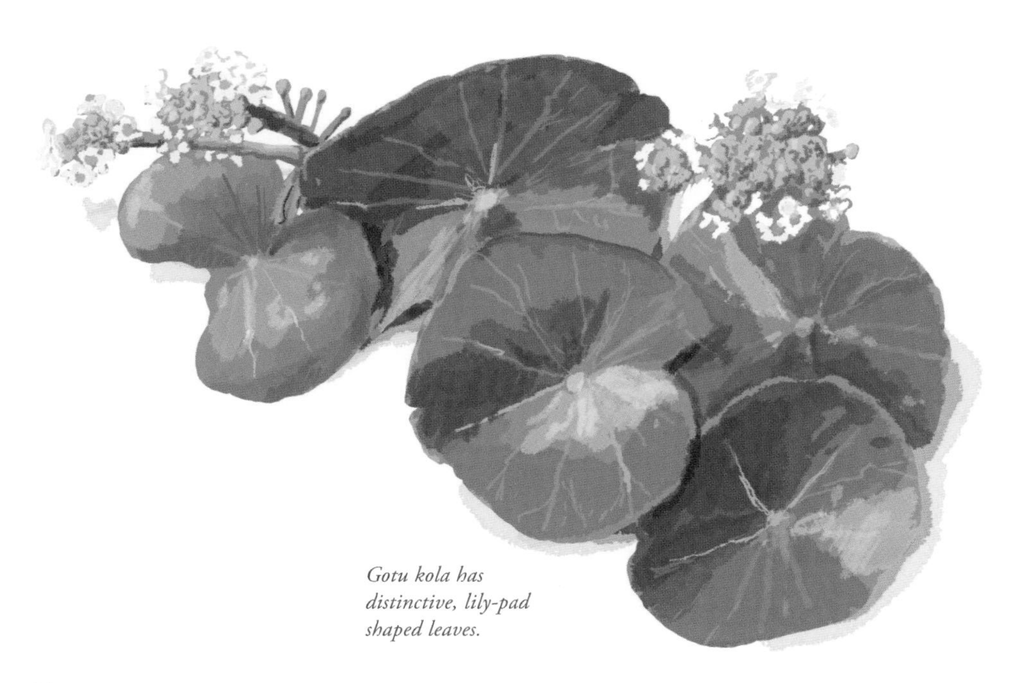

Gotu kola has distinctive, lily-pad shaped leaves.

Black Cohosh
Cimicifuga racemosa

Known as squatroot by Native Americans who used it for feminine problems, black cohosh has a stimulant effect on the uterus, so it should not be used during pregnancy. Other uses include treating bronchitis and nausea associated with headaches.

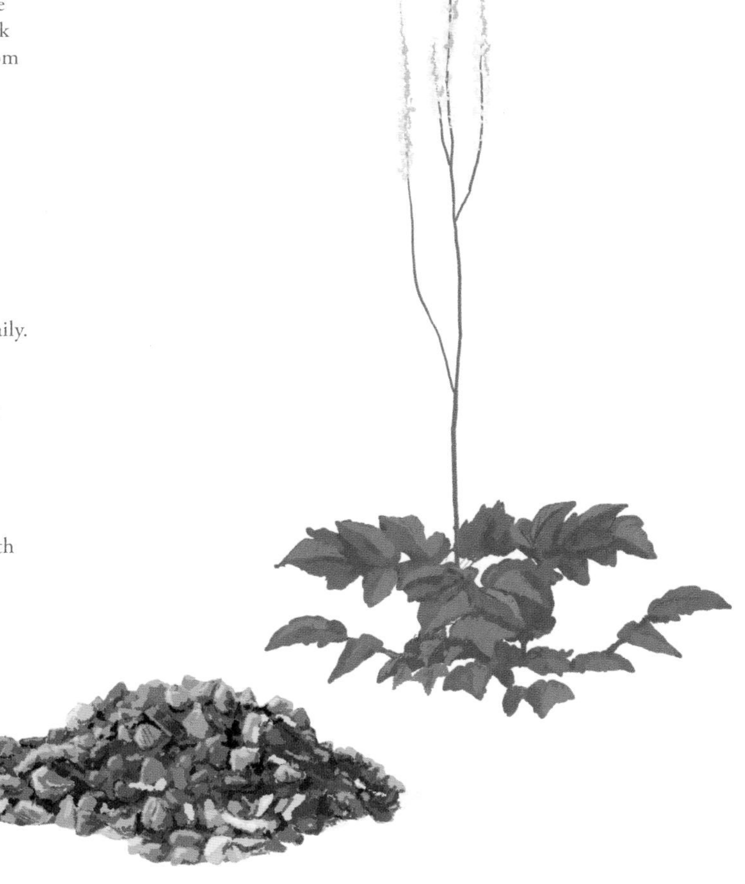

Origins & Characteristics
Black cohosh can also be used for digestive problems and to soothe arthritic aches and pains. Its use as a medicine can be traced back to a traditional Chinese text from c.A.D. 25–200.

Parts Used
Rhizome, for medicinal preparations

Dosage
Take 1 or 2 tablets (50mg) of dried herb daily. As a liquid tincture, take 20 drops twice daily.

Potential Benefits
- Reduces muscular discomfort associated with arthritis
- Calms menstrual cramps
- May be helpful in chronic bronchitis
- Reduces nausea associated with headaches

Caution
Because of the stimulant effect on the uterine muscles, avoid during pregnancy.

The root of black cohosh – dried – is the active part.

Myrrh
Commiphora molmol

Ever since biblical times, myrrh has been an essential and standard medicine used in the Middle East for the treatment of wounds, infections and digestive problems. It is especially associated with women's health and purification.

Origins & Characteristics
Myrrh has the ability to stimulate healing and reduce inflammation. Its antiseptic properties make it an effective wound cleanser. Taken internally with echinacea (*Echinacea purpura*), it can speed recovery from infections, especially chest infections, as it has good expectorant and decongestant properties. Myrrh is often taken for relieving colds and bronchitis. When used as a mouthwash myrrh can strengthen the gums and reduce gum infection and inflammation.

Parts Used
Gum resin

Dosage
As a mouthwash, add 5 drops to a little water.

As a liquid tincture, take 10 drops daily.

Potential Benefits
- Fights gum infections
- Acts as a wound-cleansing agent
- Helps fight chest infections
- Reduces bruising

Caution
Do not take myrrh in high doses during pregnancy.

Myrrh is used as a resin, made from sap drained from the tree.

Coriander
Coriandrum sativum

Coriander has been used as a culinary and medicinal herb throughout the centuries. Taken internally, this herb is used to aid digestion and to stimulate the appetite. It also reduces flatulence and helps relieve colic. The seeds are used as a spice.

Origins & Characteristics
Coriander can be especially helpful in reducing diarrhoea in children. As an external application, the lightly bruised seeds can be used as a poultice to alleviate painful joints and rheumatic symptoms.

Parts Used
Leaves and seeds

Dosage
As an infusion, add 1 teaspoon of crushed seeds to 250ml (9fl oz) of boiling water and let stand for 5 minutes. To relieve flatulence, drink before food.

For external application, use the seeds to make a poultice for painful joints.

Potential Benefits
- Aids digestion
- Stimulates the appetite
- Relieves flatulence
- Reduces diarrhoea
- Helps painful joints

Culinary Uses
Use fresh leaves on poultry dishes and add to green salads. Alternatively, use as an ingredient in salad dressings.

Chilli-and-coriander vinaigrette

You will need:
- 3 green chillies, deseeded and chopped
- ½ teaspoon ground cumin
- 3 tablespoons cider vinegar
- pinch of salt
- 125ml (4fl oz) groundnut oil
- 1 tablespoon chopped coriander leaves

Whisk together the chillies, cumin, cider vinegar and a pinch of salt. Slowly pour in the groundnut oil, whisking until well emulsified. Stir in the chopped coriander leaves before serving.

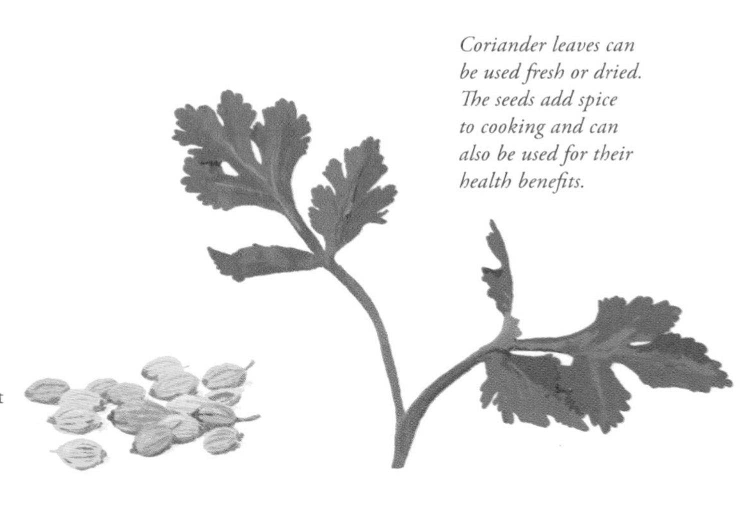

Coriander leaves can be used fresh or dried. The seeds add spice to cooking and can also be used for their health benefits.

Hawthorn
Crataegus oxyacantha

Hawthorn berries have been used by herbalists for digestive problems for many years. The berries are rich in vitamin C and bioflavonoids – essential factors for blood vessel strength and health – but it also has benefits for heart health. Its activity on the heart has been likened to that of a heart tonic.

Origins & Characteristics
The heart benefits from hawthorn in a number of ways. First, the heartbeat is strengthened, which aids a failing heart. Second, the blood vessels are dilated, which reduces the blood pressure and the resultant strain on the heart.

Hawthorn also has an effective diuretic action on the body, ridding it of the excess fluid commonly retained by those with heart problems.

Parts Used
Fruits

Dosage
As a liquid tincture, take 20 drops twice daily.

Potential Benefits
- May be used as a heart tonic
- Increases efficiency of the heartbeat
- Reduces blood pressure
- Acts as a diuretic

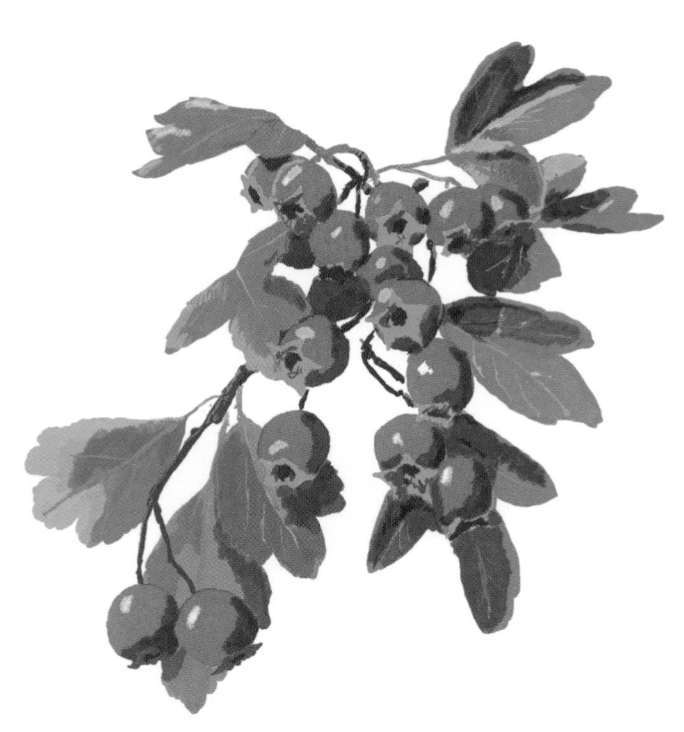

Hawthorn berries are abundant in hedgerows in late summer and autumn.

Turmeric
Curcuma longa

This is a classically pungent herb that forms the basis of most curry powders. Its ability to treat stomach problems effectively has been known for centuries in Asia but only recently in the United States and Europe. Turmeric has the ability to stimulate the flow of bile and, therefore, promote the digestion of fats effectively.

Origins & Characteristics
Turmeric has beneficial effects on the circulation, increasing peripheral distribution of blood and helping to reduce the incidence of clots. It may also help in menstrual problems, especially in congestive types of premenstrual syndrome, by helping the flow of blood.

Parts Used
Rhizome

Dosage
Take 2 tablets (50mg) of dried herb daily after eating.

Potential Benefits
- Increases circulation
- Reduces blood clots
- May help in menstrual problems
- Stimulates bile flow
- Aids in fat digestion

Culinary Uses
Forms the basis of most curries and curry powders.

It is the root of the turmeric plant that has healing properties. For cooking, it is usually dried and ground.

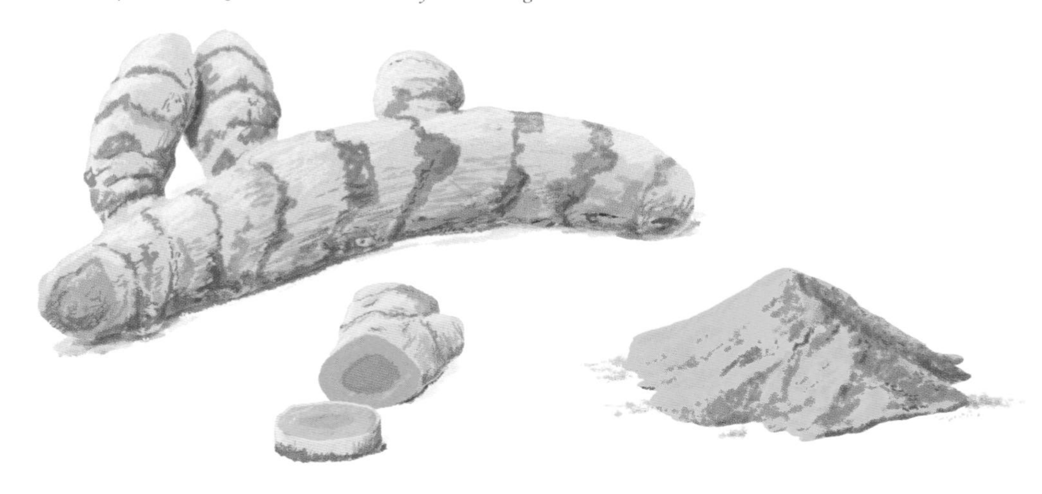

Artichoke
Cynara scolymus

Much prized by the Romans and Greeks, the artichoke has been used for medicinal purposes for centuries. The discovery of a substance called cynarin, which is contained in the leaves, supported the age-old tradition of taking artichoke for problems relating to digestion. Cynarin appears to improve the flow of bile and thus improve the liver function. A secondary effect is a reduction in cholesterol levels due to the increased flow of bile.

Parts Used
Flower heads, leaves and roots

Dosage
As a liquid tincture, take 20 drops twice daily.

Potential Benefits
- Stimulates the flow of digestive juices
- Increases bile flow
- Promotes liver function
- Reduces cholesterol levels

Culinary Uses
Artichoke vinaigrette is a delicious and sophisticated dish. Place an unopened flower head in a pan of boiling water. Reduce the heat and cook for about 15 minutes or until the leaves can be pulled off easily. Drain well, place on a small serving plate and drizzle a simple vinaigrette dressing over the leaves. Serve immediately.

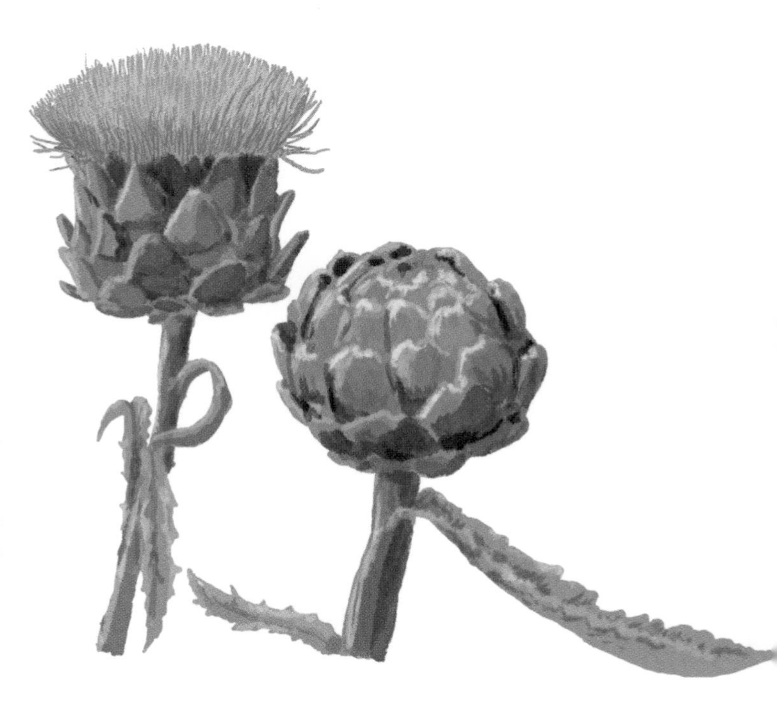

Artichokes are stately plants with striking flowerheads.

Echinacea
Echinacea purpura

The hedgehog-like appearance of the central cone of echinacea, or purple coneflower, gave this herb its name, from the Greek *echinos* meaning 'hedgehog'. Echinacea is probably one of the most commonly used herbal extracts today. In Germany, the liquid extract is referred to as 'resistance drops', owing to echinacea's immune-stimulating effect.

Parts Used
Roots and rhizomes

Dosage
In acute illness, take up to 40 drops (20 for children) of liquid tincture every four hours.

For prevention of colds and flu, take 10–15 drops daily or 1 or 2 tablets (50–100mg) of dried extract daily.

For external application, use as a cream for cuts and scrapes.

Potential Benefits
- Stimulates the immune system
- Prevents the progression of infections
- Relieves symptoms of colds and flu, especially when nasal congestion is a problem
- Has a virus killing action

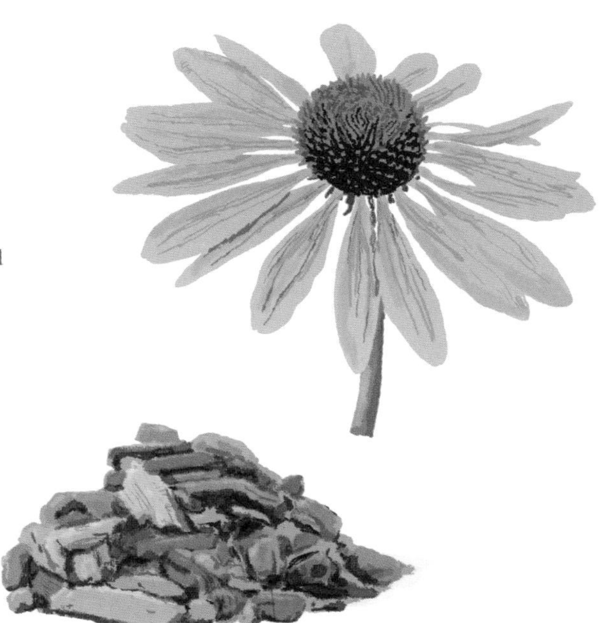

The flowers of echinacea seem to stretch up to the sun; they must be sacrificed to harvest the roots, which are dried for medicinal use.

Ginseng (Siberian)
Eleutherococcus senticosus

The active agents of Siberian ginseng are similar to the *Panax* ginseng form (page 92) but are considered to be less potent. Siberian ginseng can be taken for longer periods than *Panax* ginseng and is thought to be better suited to the treatment of stress when an extended treatment programme is needed.

Origins & Characteristics
As well as its benefits for people suffering from stress, Siberian ginseng may also be used to improve physical and mental stamina. There are claims that it may reduce cholesterol and blood sugar levels.

Parts Used
Roots

Dosage
Take 2 teaspoons of ginseng elixir daily.

Potential Benefits
- Improves resistance to stress
- Increases mental agility
- May reduce cholesterol and blood sugar levels

Caution
Generally, Siberian ginseng should not be used continuously for longer than one month.

Ginseng roots can be used to make a healing elixir.

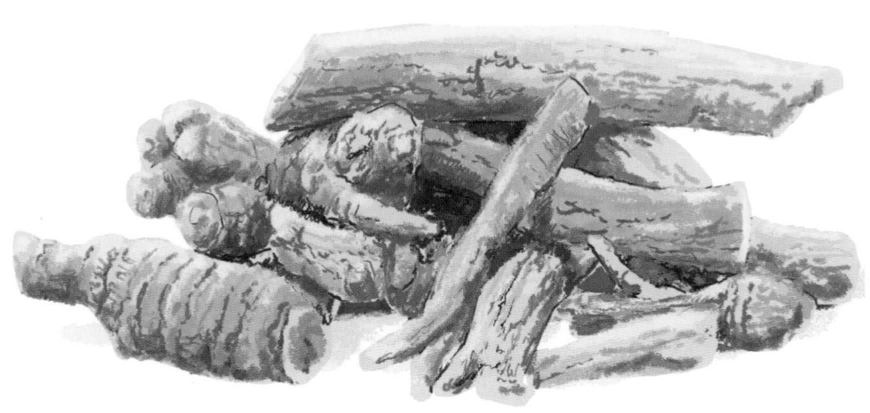

Horsetail
Equisetum arvense

Contained within this herb is an interesting cocktail of nutrients and phytochemicals. Horsetail is rich in silica and other minerals that facilitate the absorption of calcium from the diet, and this high silica content may make it helpful in reducing cholesterol levels.

Origins & Characteristics
Because of its role in helping the body to absorb calcium, nails and hair greatly benefit from this herb, as do the bones and other connective tissues that depend on calcium and trace minerals for their health.

Parts Used
Stems

Dosage
As a liquid tincture, take 15–20 drops twice daily.

Potential Benefits
- Adds strength to nails and hair
- Supports healthy bone and tissue development
- Helps reduce acne in those with oily skin
- May help reduce cholesterol levels

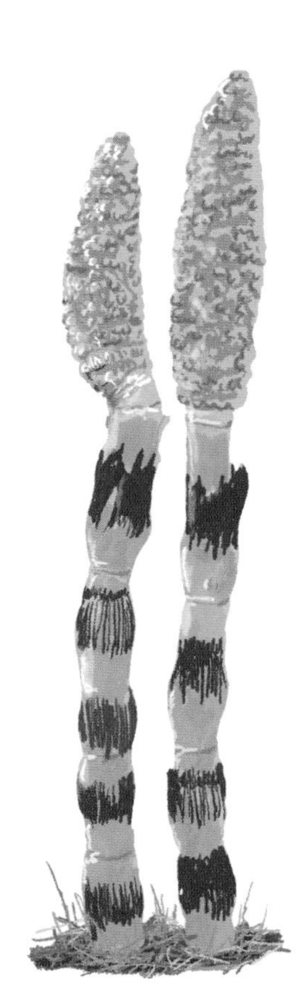

The distinctive stripy stems of horsetail are rich in silica.

Californian Poppy
Eschscholzia californica

The watery sap of this plant has a mild painkilling action. The Native Americans often used this to reduce the pain of toothache. It has also been used as a sedative and may help insomnia.

Origins & Characteristics
The painkilling action of the Californian poppy appears to work on the body's central nervous system and is thought to be narcotic in nature.

Parts Used
Whole plant

Dosage
As a liquid tincture, take 5–10 drops as needed.

Potential Benefits
- Has a painkilling action if applied topically in cases of toothache
- Reduces anxiety and tension when used internally
- May help insomnia

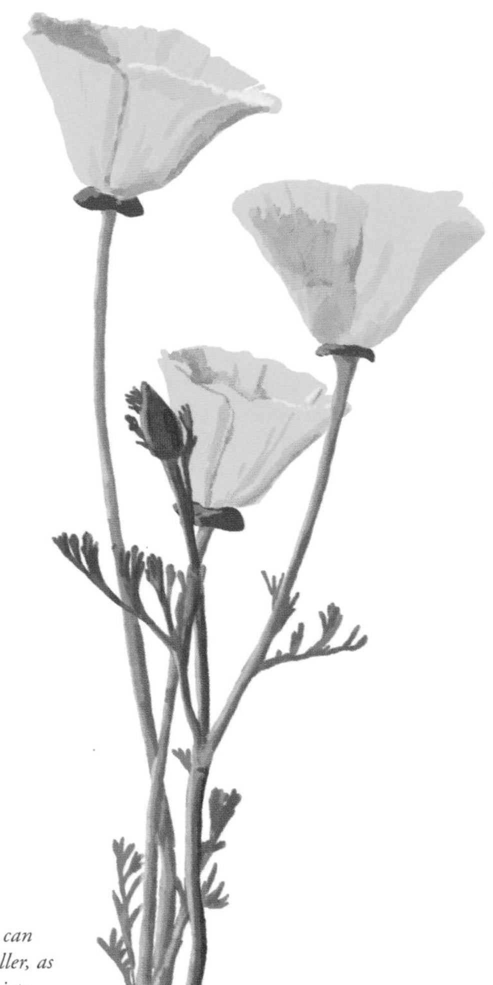

The Californian poppy can act as a natural painkiller, as well as combatting anxiety.

Eucalyptus
Eucalyptus globulus

There are more than 40 different types of eucalyptus trees, all of which are rich in the volatile oils that are responsible for the distinctive aroma. Traditional aboriginal uses are well-kept secrets, but it was known to help treat dysentery.

Origins & Characteristics

The extracts from eucalyptus have a great decongestant action due to the high content of aromatic oils, and it is for this property that the plant is best known. Eucalyptus, also called the blue gum tree, can help in expectoration because it acts as a respiratory stimulant.

Used externally, eucalyptus can help to heal sports injuries. Eucalyptus has an antiseptic action that helps to reduce muscle spasm. Muscular aches and pains benefit greatly from an application of a eucalyptus-based cream or lotion.

Parts Used

Leaves and essential oils

Dosage

As a vapor inhalant, use about 4 drops in a vaporizer and inhale for about 5 minutes.

For external application, use as a cream or lotion, as required.

Potential Benefits

- Acts as a decongestant for upper respiratory infections
- Clears sinus congestion
- Stimulates the removal of lung congestion
- Has an antimicrobial activity
- Can be used as an effective muscle ointment

Cosmetic Uses

Can be used in a lotion or skin tonic to stimulate the skin's circulation. Add a couple of drops of essential oil to a bath to soothe aching muscles.

Caution

Do not use on open wounds. Avoid excessive exposure to vapours, as eucalyptus can cause headaches and may aggravate asthma symptoms.

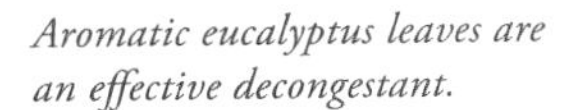

Aromatic eucalyptus leaves are an effective decongestant.

Eyebright
Euphrasis officinalis

The *Doctrine of Signatures* – an ancient herbal text – purports that if the appearance of a plant or flower looks like an anatomical part, then the herb will help diseases of that area. By this doctrine, eyebright became a cure-all for eye problems – the flowers have purple and yellow stripes and spots that resemble the human iris.

Origins & Characteristics
The astringent properties of eyebright make it a useful herb for the treatment of sore and inflamed eyes (conjunctivitis) and other irritant eye problems, such as weeping eczema, which can occur around the eyes, as well as ultra-sensitivity to light.

Parts Used
Whole plant

Dosage
For an eye bath, use a commercially made preparation to minimise the risk of infection.

As a liquid tincture, take 1 or 2 drops twice daily.

Potential Benefits
- Calms irritated eyes and helps reduce conjunctivitis
- Promotes good eye health when taken internally

Caution
Avoid high doses of eyebright during pregnancy.

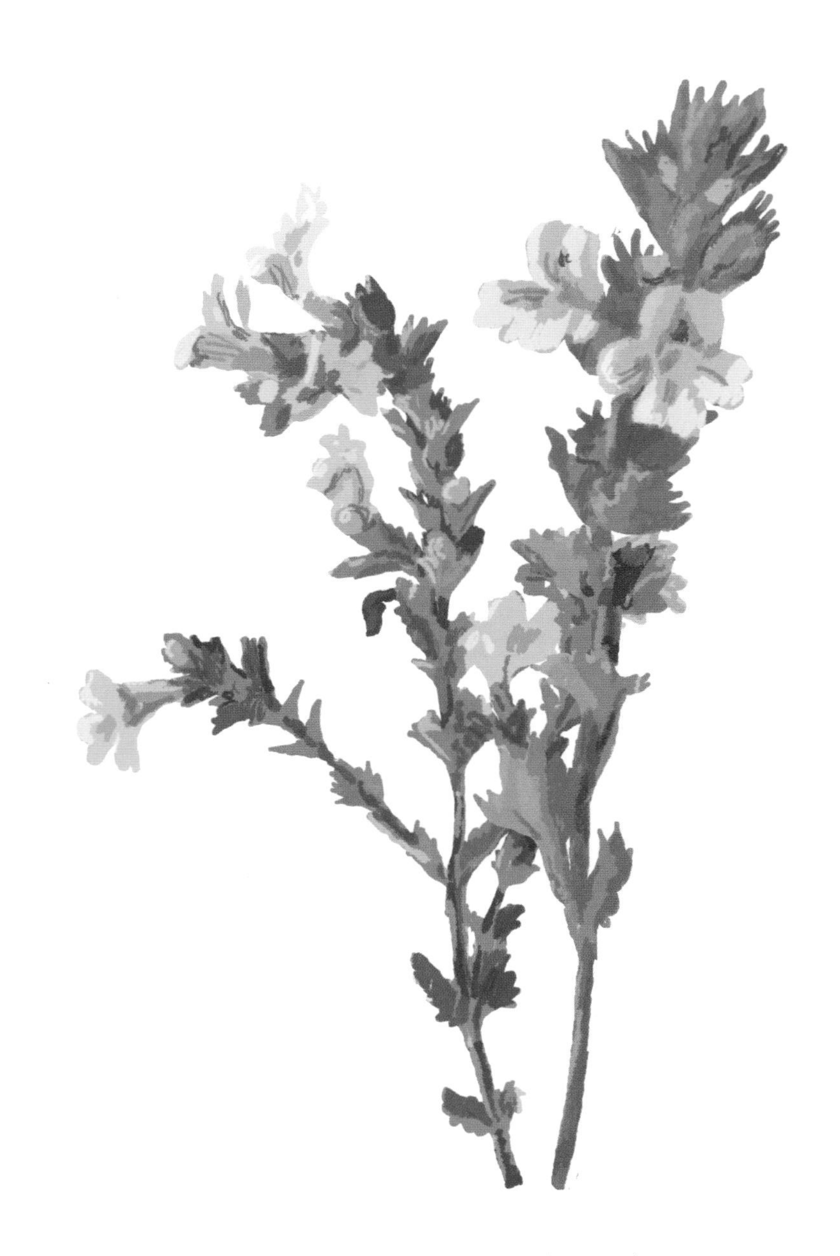

A resemblance in the flowers to the markings of the human iris gave eyebright its common name.

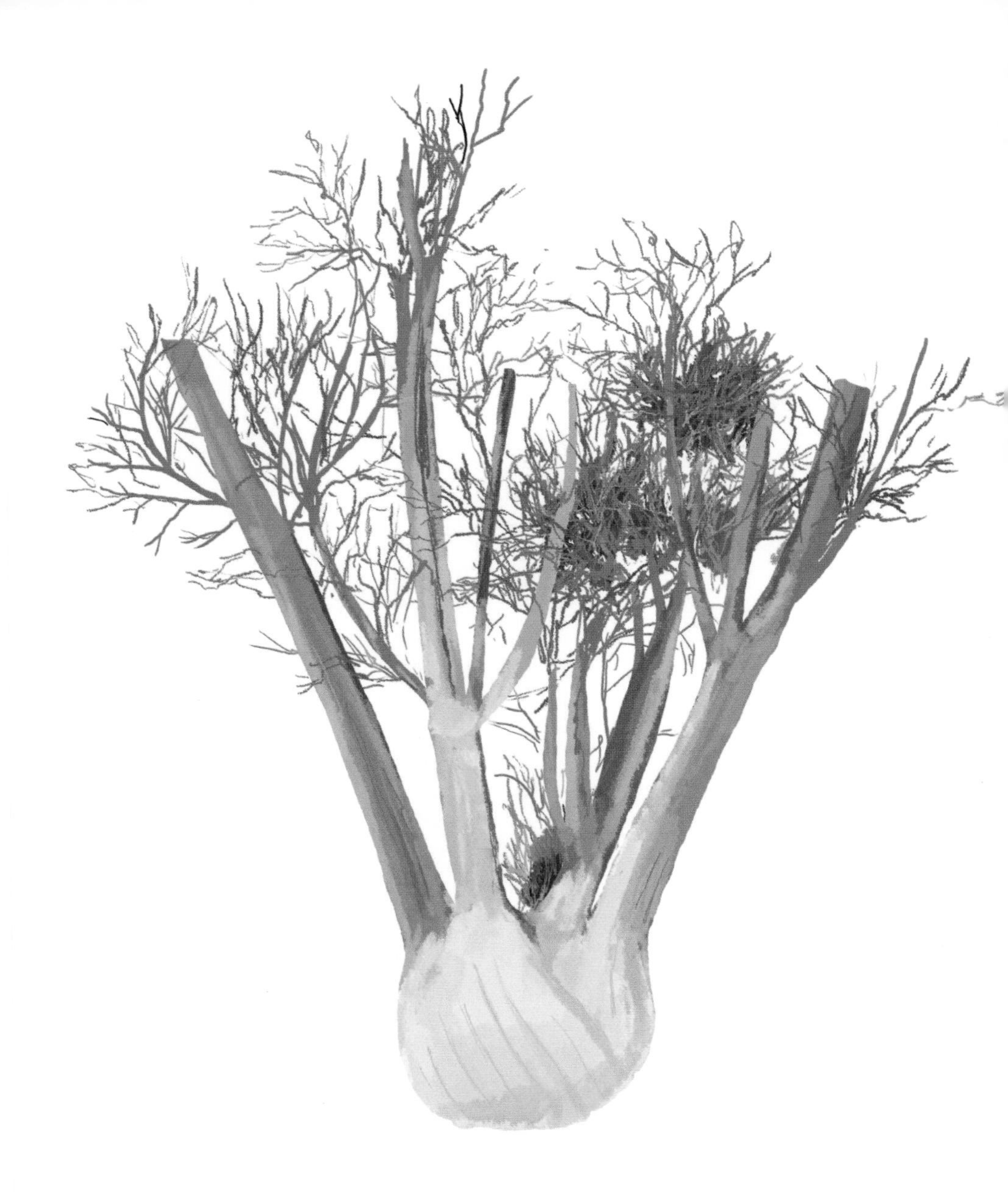

Fennel leaves can be used for flavour in cooking, or the bulb itself can be cooked and eaten as a vegetable.

Fennel
Foeniculum vulgare

Fresh fennel delivers a special aroma due to the two oils, anethole and fenchone, which vary from species to species. Taken internally, fennel aids the digestive process and soothes cases of colic and abdominal discomfort.

Origins & Characteristics
Fennel can be taken as a tea or as 'fennel water', which is very easy to make, but is sold for babies as gripe water. If drunk during breastfeeding it may help to reduce colic in the infant. Fennel also has a mild diuretic action and a cleansing action on the kidneys and it is thought to promote the flow of breast milk in nursing mothers.

Parts Used
Leaves, stems, roots and seeds

Dosage
As a liquid tincture, take 20 drops just after eating. As fennel water, put about 2 pinches of fennel seeds in 250ml (9fl oz) of water and bring to a boil. As the water starts to change colour, keep boiling for 1 minute. Strain and cool before drinking. Keep in the fridge.

As a tea, add 2 teaspoons of seeds to 250ml (9fl oz) of boiling water and steep for 5 minutes.

Potential Benefits
- Acts as a digestive aid
- Reduces abdominal cramping and colic
- Reduces flatulence
- Acts as a remedy for infantile colic
- Acts as a mild diuretic and kidney cleanser
- Promotes flow of breast milk in nursing mothers

Cosmetic Uses
The seeds can be used in a lotion to help oily skin.

Culinary Uses
Try fennel seeds in fish dishes or use during the cooking of vegetables. Fresh fennel bulb can be cooked whole and eaten as a vegetable.

Fennel has a wonderful aniseed flavour and is a good accompaniment to poultry and lamb dishes.

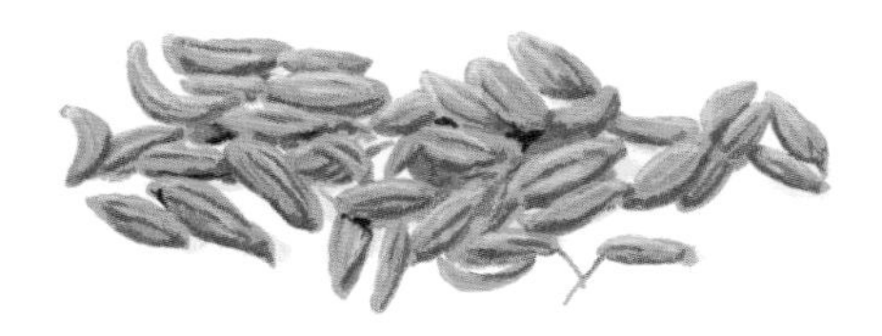

Fennel seeds are useful for flavouring, but also make a tea that can aid digestion.

American Cranesbill
Geranium maculatum

This herb is known to be a common medicine used by Native Americans for the treatment of diarrhoea and stomach complaints. Another traditional use of this plant is the control of excessive bleeding associated with menstruation, but it is also useful in the treatment of infection.

Origins & Characteristics
Analysis of the plant extracts shows a high concentration of astringents. A topical application of the plant is used to treat infected wounds, thrush and haemorrhoids.

Parts Used
Whole plant

Dosage
As a liquid tincture, take 20–25 drops twice daily.
For external application, use as a compress for wounds, thrush and haemorrhoids.

Potential Benefits
- Has an antiseptic action
- Reduces blood flow in menstruation
- Soothes haemorrhoid irritation
- Reduces diarrhoea

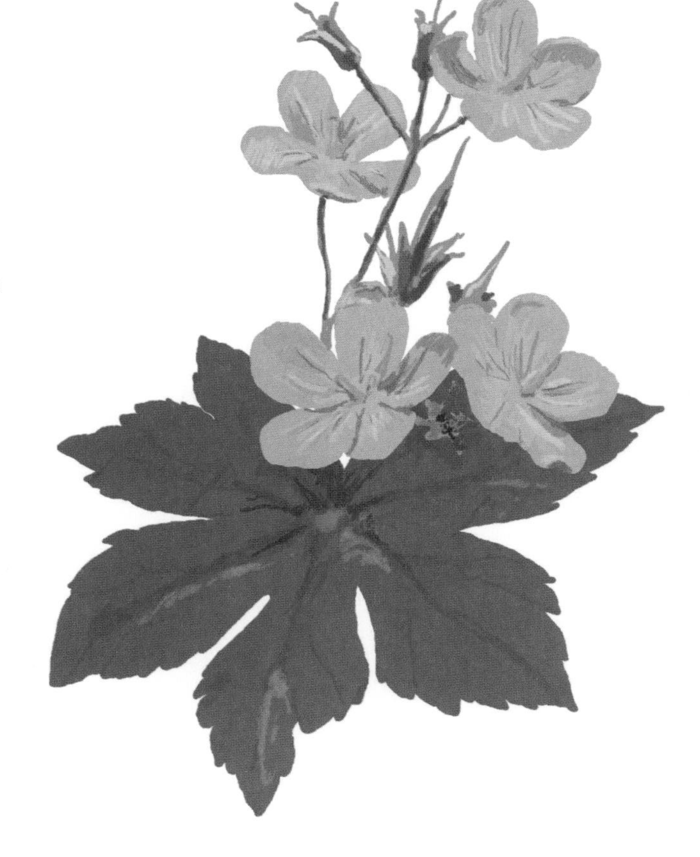

The American cranesbill is sometimes known as geranium. It is a pretty garden perennial plant.

Ginkgo
Ginkgo biloba

Fossil records show that the ginkgo tree has remained unchanged for millions of years. The trees were present even before mammals walked the earth. Ginkgo is one of the most well-known and popular herbal remedies and is particularly useful in the treatment of allergies.

Origins & Characteristics

Extracts of the leaves of the ginkgo plant yield a fascinating substance that has profound effects on the allergic response. These chemicals, ginkgolides, act to inhibit platelet-activating factor, a key substance in the allergic response. Other chemicals, ginkgo flavonoids, have a stimulating effect on the blood circulation of the brain and periphery.

Ginkgo has been effectively used for the treatment of asthma, tinnitus, allergic inflammatory conditions and varicose veins. It has also been used to treat reduced brain circulation and Raynaud's disease, as this herb improves peripheral circulation. In this disease, peripheral circulation is badly affected, and the hands often turn blue.

Parts Used

Leaves and seeds

Dosage

As a liquid tincture, take 20 drops twice daily.

Potential Benefits

- Improves blood circulation to the brain
- Reduces symptoms of tinnitus
- Reduces allergic conditions
- Helps in Raynaud's disease
- May reduce asthma symptoms

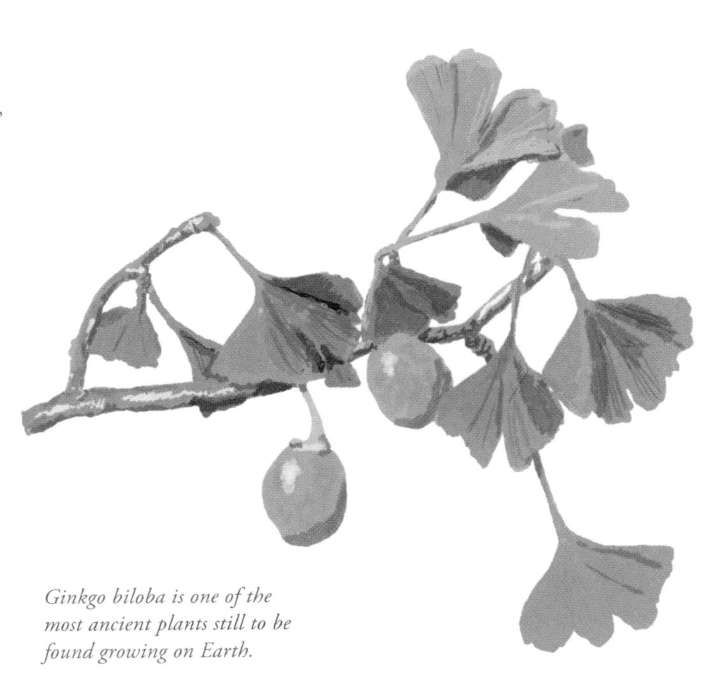

Ginkgo biloba is one of the most ancient plants still to be found growing on Earth.

Licorice
Glycyrrhiza glabra

The main constituent of licorice is a substance called glycyrrhizin, which is 50 times sweeter than sugar. Glycyrrhizin reduces inflammation and has been used in treating menstrual irregularities. Taken 14 days prior to menstruation, licorice can suppress the breakdown of progesterone and improve depression, sugar cravings, water retention and breast tenderness.

Origins & Characteristics
Taken internally, licorice can help Addison's disease, as glycyrrhizin has a similar effect to an adrenal hormone called aldosterone. Licorice has a detoxifying action on the liver.

An oestrogen-like action has been noted, making it a good remedy for the relief of menopausal symptoms. Taken for stomach problems, licorice has a great healing power on the lining of the stomach.

Parts Used
Roots

Dosage
Chew 2 or 3 tablets (100mg) with each meal.

Potential Benefits
- Speeds the healing of stomach ulcers
- Helps in menstrual irregularities
- Detoxifies the liver
- Helps in Addison's disease
- Relieves the symptoms of the menopause

Caution
Because of the sodium content of licorice avoid taking it during pregnancy. Do not use if you have high blood pressure or kidney disease or if you are taking the heart drug Digoxin.

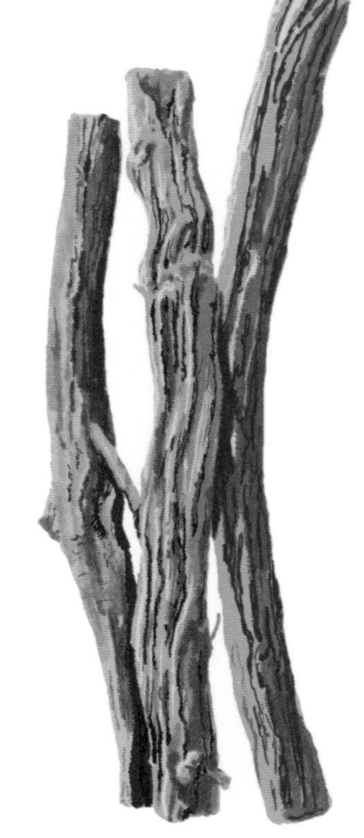

Licorice root can be chewed in its dried form or taken as a tablet. Even the candied form – Pontefract cakes – can be helpful.

Hop
Humulus lupulus

Hops are one of nature's best relaxants. The herb exerts a calming effect on the whole body, relieving nervous tension, irritability and insomnia. For the treatment of irritable bowel syndrome and a nervous stomach, hops can prove to be a very effective remedy. A good combination is equal parts of valerian (*Valeriana officinalis*) and hops taken about a half hour before bed to induce a natural and restful sleep.

Parts Used
Leaves and shoots

Dosage
As a soothing agent for irritable bowels, take 2 tablets (50mg) of hops daily.
As a sedative, try the mixture described in the introduction above at bedtime.
For external application, use as a poultice for eczema and skin ulcers.

Potential Benefits
- Acts as a sedative to promote restful sleep
- Acts as a calming agent for a nervous stomach
- Relieves irritable bowel syndrome
- Acts as an anti-stress herb
- Relieves eczema and skin ulcerations

Culinary Uses
The young side shoots can be cooked and eaten.

Caution
Avoid if you suffer from depression.

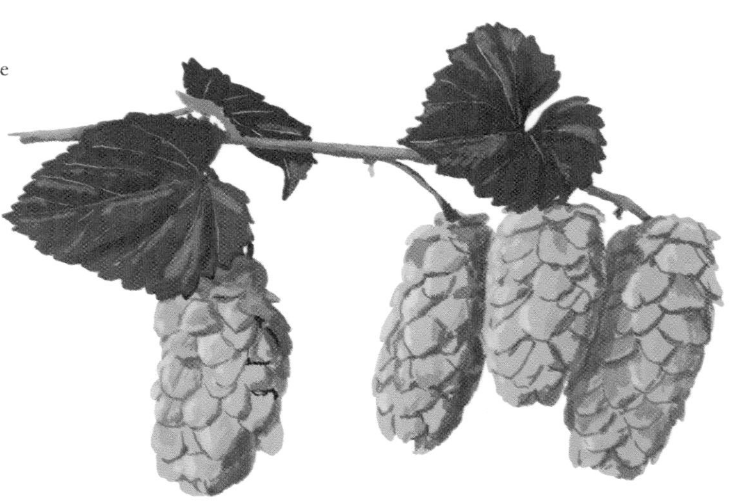

Hops have excellent calming properties, useful to relieve nervous tension.

Goldenseal
Hydrastis canadensis

Goldenseal can act as a double-edged sword. When given for infections of the bowels, it tends to destroy the beneficial bacteria as well as the disease-causing ones. It is recommended, therefore, that its use should be restricted to one month followed by a course of probiotics – capsules containing cultures of good bacteria for the bowel.

Origins & Characteristics
Goldenseal can also be used as a laxative. Externally, it can be used for treating irritated skin and conjunctivitis.

Parts Used
Rhizomes

Dosage
As a liquid tincture, take 20 drops daily.

For an eyebath to relieve the symptoms of conjunctivitis, use a commercially made preparation to minimise the risk of infection.

For external application, use as a lotion, compress or cream and apply as required.

Potential Benefits
- Reduces constipation
- Has an antibacterial action in bowel and gut infections
- Helps relieve irritated skin
- Acts as a laxative

Caution
Do not use for longer than one month. Avoid during pregnancy as goldenseal stimulates the uterine muscles.

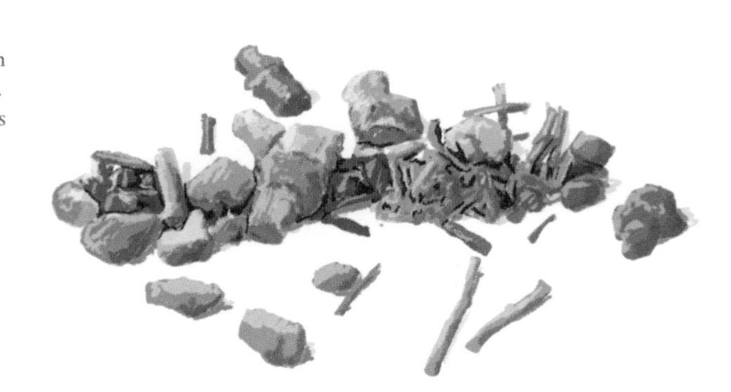

There are few ailments that goldsenseal has not at some time been used to treat. The roots are dried and chopped, then powdered before use.

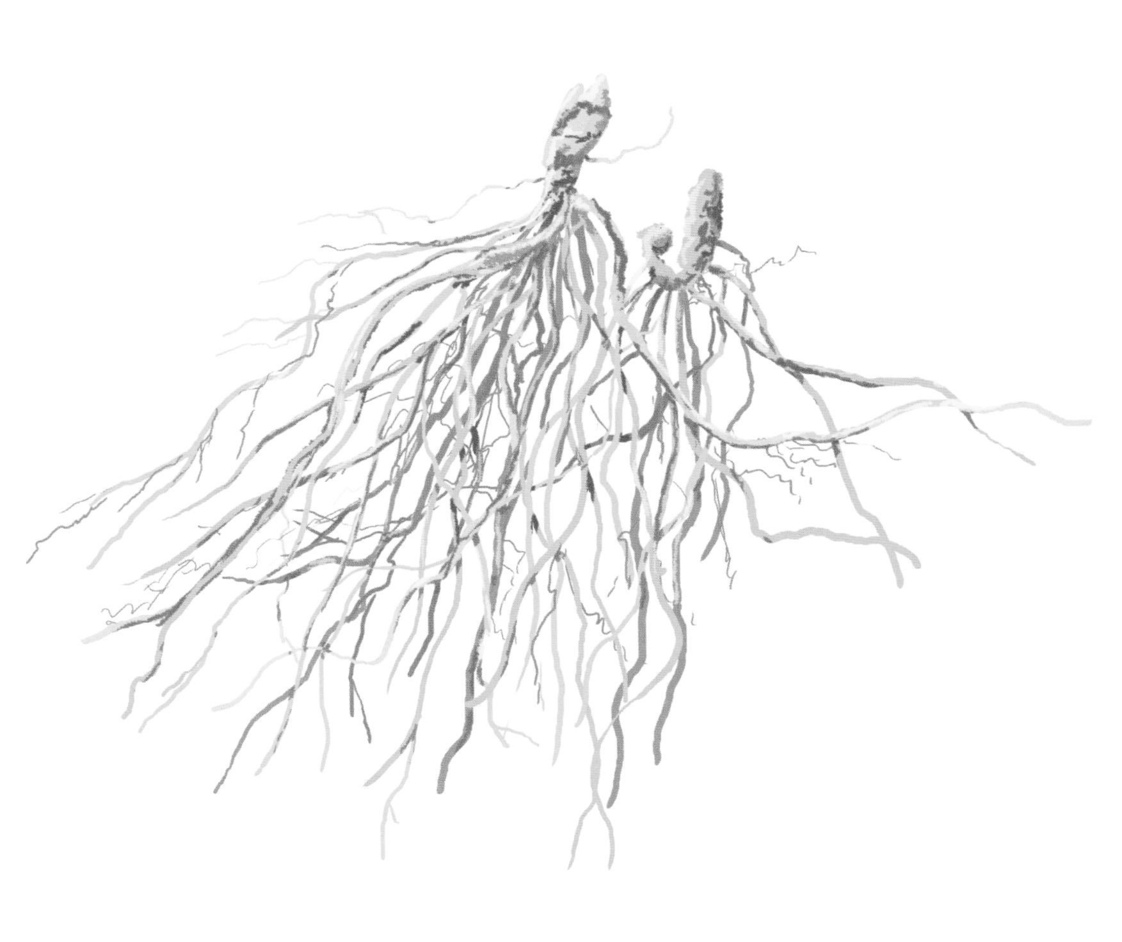

Goldenseal is a member of the buttercup family. Its bright golden roots have myriad uses, but it must be taken with caution.

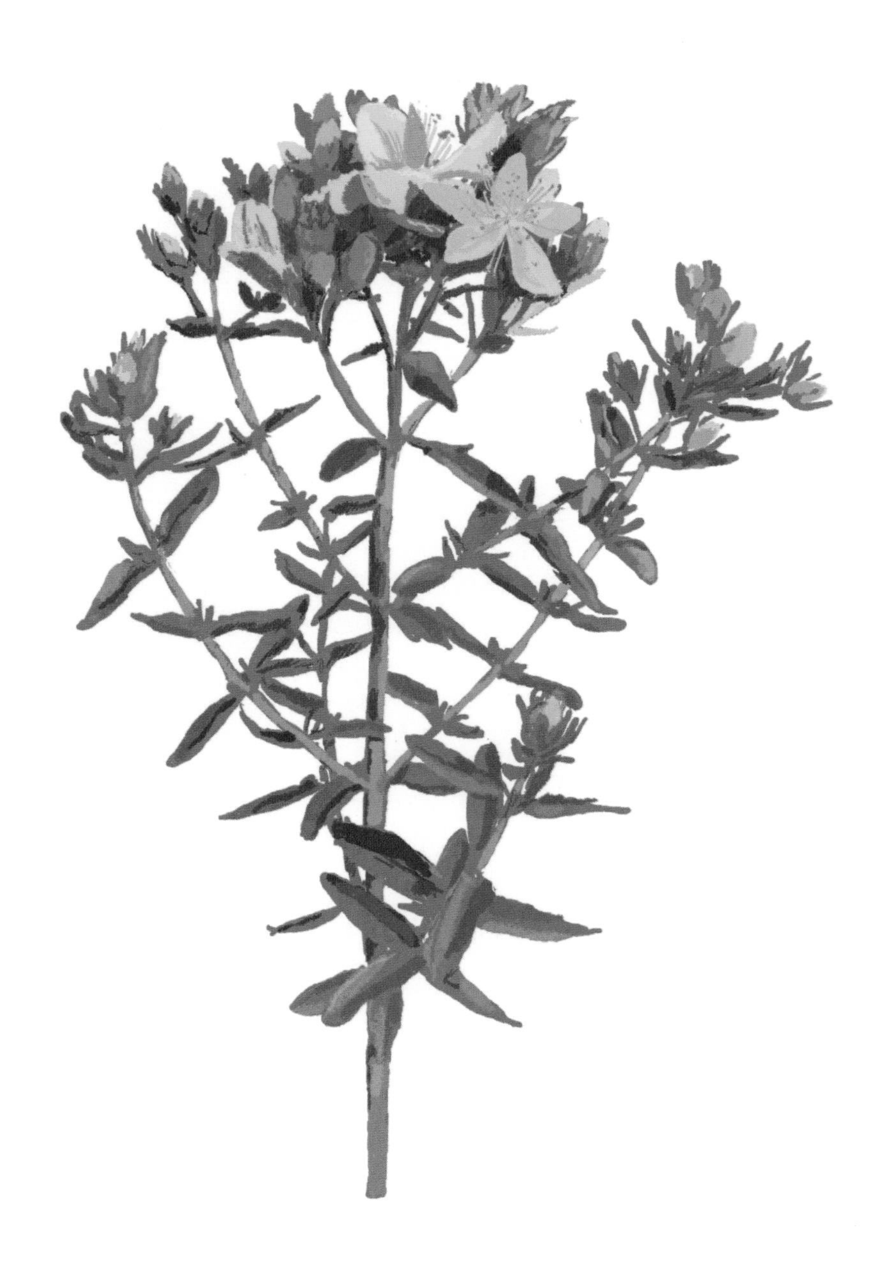

St. John's Wort is well known as a treatment for depression, but also helps to treat wounds.

St. John's Wort
Hypericum perfortum

There has been much interest in this herb since a study found it to be as effective as regular anti-depressants, but with none of the accompanying side effects. St. John's wort has an effective sedative action and can calm nerves and help relieve insomnia.

Origins & Characteristics
The effective anti-depressant action was found to be due to the high concentration of hypericin. This herb produces a lovely red pigment when the leaves are crushed between the fingers, and it is the pigment that contains the active agents.

Another interesting aspect to this herb is its ability to stop the multiplication of certain viruses (retroviruses), meaning it may be used to treat AIDS.

Used externally as a lotion, St. John's wort has a powerful healing and anti-inflammatory action and can be used to treat varicose veins, bruises and painful sunburn.

Parts Used
Whole plant

Dosage
As a liquid tincture, take 20 drops twice daily.

For external application, use as a lotion as required.

Potential Benefits
- Acts as a remedy for insomnia
- Calms nerves
- Promotes wound-healing
- Has a potential benefit against AIDS
- Relieves sunburn

Hyssop
Hyssopus officinalis

Hyssop is mentioned in the New Testament of the Bible as an herb that has purification properties. These are largely due to the high content of camphoraceous oils contained within the herb. Its effectiveness in treating lung infections, such as bronchitis, can be attributed to this substance. It can also be used to relieve coughs, colds and nasal congestion as well as making an effective gargle for sore throats.

Origins & Characteristics

Hyssop has the ability to stabilise low blood pressure and prevent the dizzy spells experienced by people with low blood pressure as they rise from a sitting or lying position.

An external application can be used for the treatment of minor cuts and bruises.

Parts Used

Whole plant

Dosage

In tablet form, take 2 tablets (50mg) of dried herb twice daily.

As a liquid tincture, take 15–20 drops twice daily.

For external application, use as a compress for minor cuts and bruises.

Potential Benefits

- Stabilises low blood pressure
- Acts against lung infections
- Helps relieve coughs
- Helps as a topical application for minor cuts and bruises

Culinary Uses

Try adding a few leaves to meat dishes including beef casseroles. It is also ideal for adding to many legume dishes.

Caution

The essential oil must be avoided during pregnancy and by people who suffer from epilepsy.

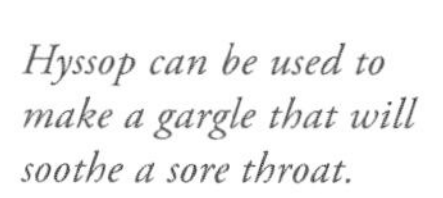

Hyssop can be used to make a gargle that will soothe a sore throat.

Jasmine
Jasmine officinale

Initially grown for the perfume industry, jasmine has many possible health-promoting effects. Jasmine has been successfully used for the treatment of sunstroke, fever, irritant dermatitis and infectious illness including coughs. Emotional upsets, postnatal depression, premenstrual tension and headaches all respond well to a dose of jasmine as it exhibits powerful anti-depressant properties.

Origins & Characteristics
Jasmine is very useful for relieving menstrual cramps, as it has the ability to reduce muscular spasms of the uterus. It is regarded as an aphrodisiac when applied to the body in its oil form.

Parts Used
Roots, flowers and oil

Dosage
As a tea, drink 1 cup of jasmine tea daily.

For external application, use 6 drops of essential oil mixed with 2 teaspoons of almond oil.

Potential Benefits
- Improves emotional state
- May help reduce dermatitis symptoms
- May act as an aphrodisiac

Cosmetic Uses
Add 6–8 drops of essential oil for a stimulating bath.

Caution
Avoid during early pregnancy.

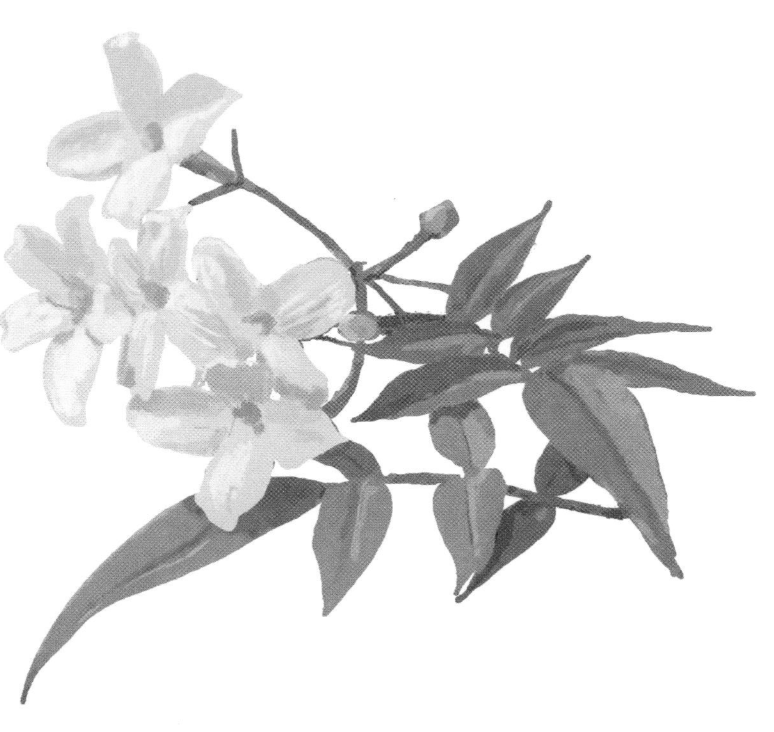

Jasmine has a strongly perfumed fragrance, often strongest in the early evening.

Juniper
Juniperus communis

Gin flavoured with juniper berries was created in the 1500s as a diuretic medicine, since it was not expensive to produce. For as long as records have been kept, juniper's diuretic action has been noted and used in the treatment of cystitis, inflammation of the kidneys, gout and arthritis.

Origins & Characteristics
An external application can be helpful for arthritis and rheumatism symptoms. Juniper is also thought to be useful in helping treat oily skin and acne.

Parts Used
Fruits

Dosage
As a liquid tincture, take 20 drops twice daily.

For external application, use 6 drops of juniper berry essential oil in 2 teaspoons of almond oil and massage into arthritic joints.

Potential Benefits
- Acts as a powerful diuretic
- Reduces symptoms of gout
- Aids in cystitis
- Soothes joint pains associated with arthritis

Cosmetic Uses
May be used in a lotion for oily skin and acne.

Culinary Uses
Add some berries to pâtés, relish or sauerkraut.

Caution
Avoid during pregnancy because of the stimulant effect on the muscles of the uterus.

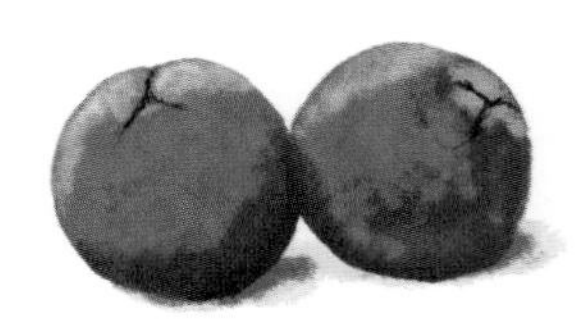

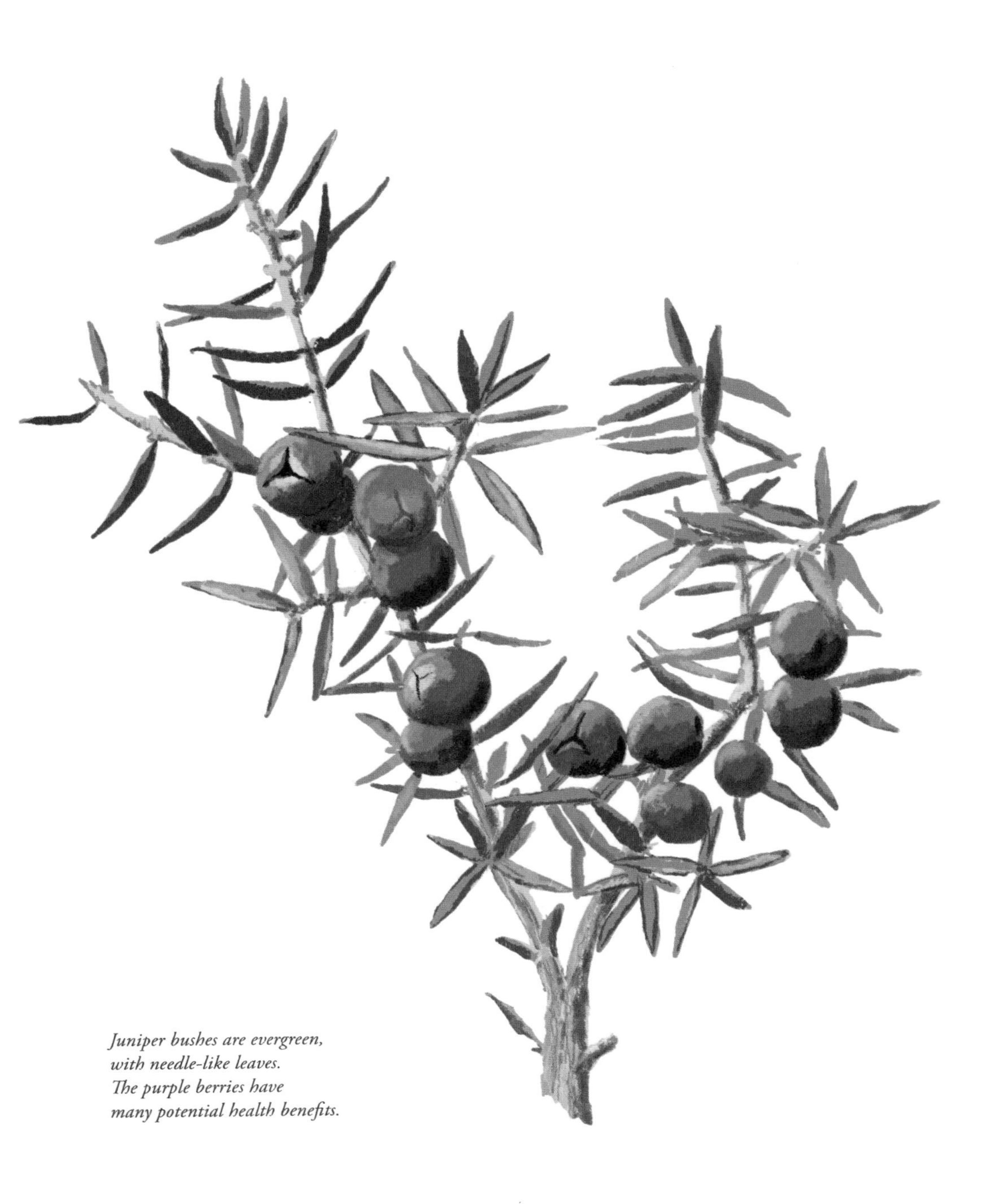

Juniper bushes are evergreen,
with needle-like leaves.
The purple berries have
many potential health benefits.

Lavender
Lavandula officinalis

The aromatic, sweet smell of lavender is unmistakable, and it is said to have anti-depressant and mood-elevating effects. As it exhibits powerful sedative and calming properties, lavender has been used for the treatment of digestive problems, anxiety, rheumatism, irritability, insomnia and tension headaches. It has also been found effective for use in migraine headaches.

Origins & Characteristics
Lavender can be used to treat minor burns, especially sunburn, and rheumatic muscular aches and pains. It is also useful in treating skin problems such as acne. Lavender is one of the most popular essential oils used for relaxation.

Parts Used
Flowers, stems and essential oil

Dosage
For external application, use 6 drops of essential oil mixed with 2 teaspoons of almond oil to treat the affected area.

For a relaxing tea, infuse a commercially prepared tea and drink twice daily.

Potential Benefits
- Has natural anti-depressant effects
- Acts as a mood lifter
- Reduces anxiety
- Helps digestion
- Soothes rheumatic muscle and joint pains
- May help relieve migraine headaches

Cosmetic Uses
Lavender may be used in a lotion for sunburn or in a cream for dry skin. Add 6–8 drops of lavender essential oil for a relaxing bath.

Culinary Uses
Try flavouring preserves with lavender or incorporating it into cake and biscuit mixes.

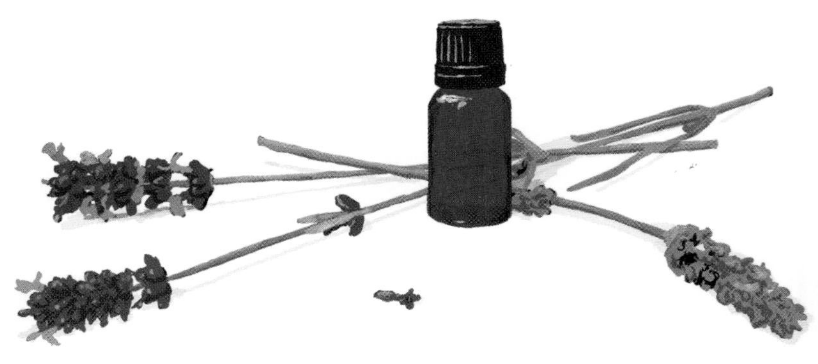

Use lavender essential oil for relaxation.

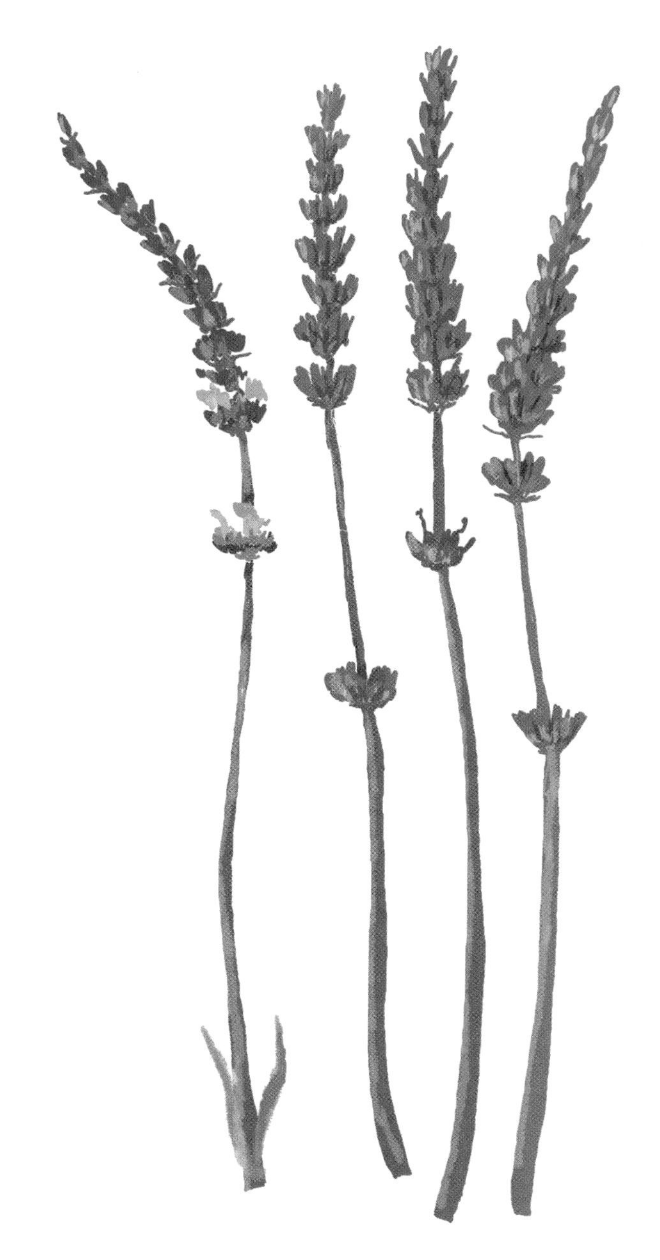

A small bag of lavender flowerheads tucked inside a pillowcase can help you to get to sleep.

Linseed or Common Flax
Linum usitatissimum

Linseed is grown as a farm crop, but contained within the plant are a number of important substances. The oil in the seeds, combined with the plant mucilage, makes an effective laxative. Linseed oil on its own has great potential to help reduce the irritation of eczema as it contains high concentrations of essential fatty acids that are needed by the skin. Externally, the crushed seeds can be used in a poultice for treating boils and pleurisy.

Parts Used
Seeds

Dosage
As a laxative, chew and swallow 1 or 2 teaspoons of seeds at bedtime with a glass of water. In cases of skin irritation, take 1 or 2g of linseed oil daily after meals.

For external application, use as a poultice made from the crushed seeds to treat boils and the symptoms of pleurisy. Apply to the painful area.

Potential Benefits
- Has laxative properties, helpful in chronic constipation
- Has an anti-inflammatory action, especially in skin problems such as eczema
- Relieves boils

Culinary Uses
Flax flour can be obtained from health food stores and makes great bread.

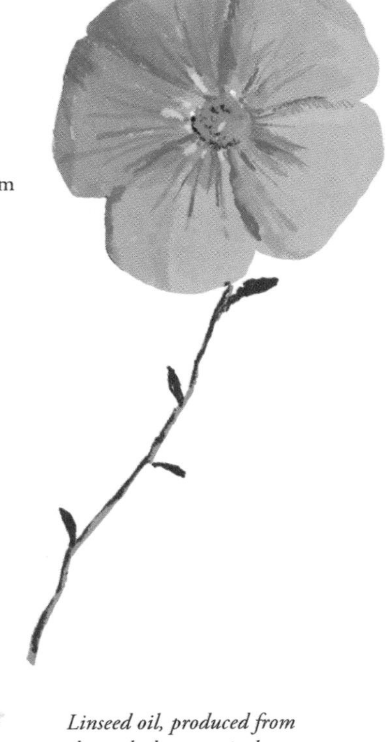

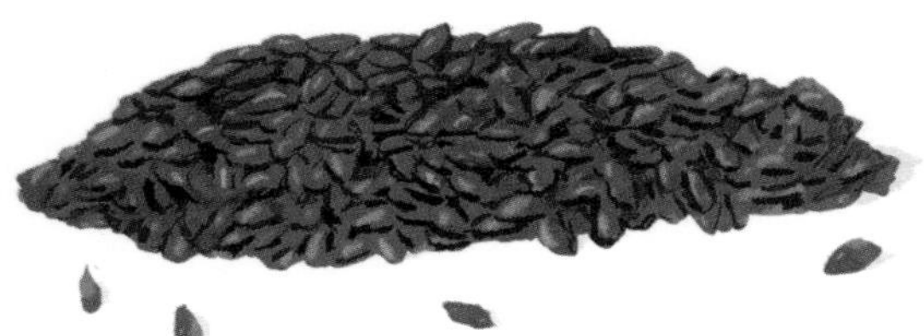

Linseed oil, produced from the seeds, has practical uses to treat and preserve wood, as well as medicinal properties.

Devil's Claw
Martynia annua

An extract of this herb is used in rural South Africa, where the locals have been long been finding relief from the symptoms of arthritis and rheumatism by drinking a decoction made from the roots of the plant. The analgesic effect of this herb is accompanied by its anti-inflammatory action, making it the herb of choice for inflammatory joint problems such as arthritis. The herb has also been noted as a digestive stimulant.

Parts Used
Tubers

Dosage
As a liquid tincture, take 20 drops twice daily.

Potential Benefits
- Has a natural painkilling anti-inflammatory action
- Soothes symptoms of arthritis and joint swelling
- Acts as a mild digestive stimulant

Caution
Avoid during pregnancy.

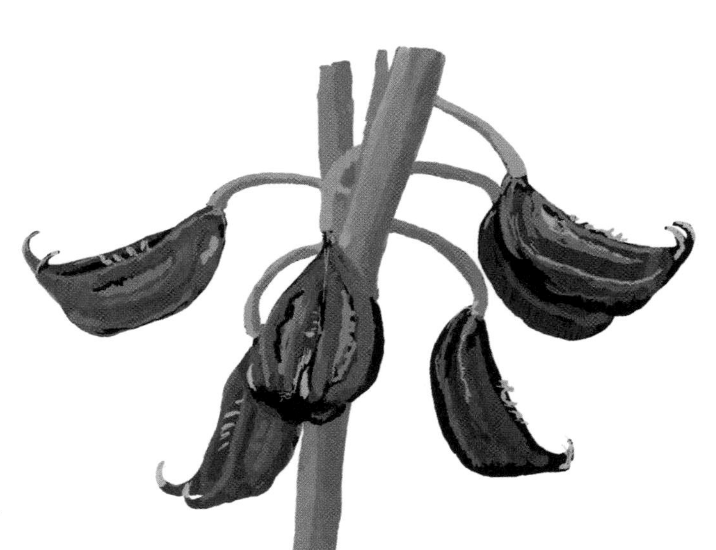

Devil's claw gets its name from the fruits, which have hooks that attach to animals' fur for seed dispersal.

Alfalfa
Medicago sativa

Alfalfa is an incredible plant. It can grow in very harsh conditions and transform barren land into a lush pasture. The nutrient content of alfalfa is impressive, comprising vitamins C, D, E, K and the B complex, as well as beta carotene and the minerals potassium, magnesium and calcium.

Origins & Characteristics

Alfalfa is a good laxative and mild diuretic and is used for urinary tract infections. It is given as a tonic for those recovering from any debilitating illness that leaves the patient weak. It has the ability to stimulate the appetite.

There can be a tendency to consume too much of this herb, but care needs to be taken because it can trigger a flare-up of systemic lupus erythematosus as well as making some people sensitive to sunlight.

Parts Used

Whole plant

Dosage

In tablet form, take up to 5 tablets of dried, compressed alfalfa plant daily.

As a liquid tincture, take 15–20 drops twice daily.

Potential Benefits

- Acts as a diuretic
- Has a laxative effect
- Helps recovery from any debilitating illness
- Helps relieve the symptoms of cystitis
- Stimulates the appetite

Culinary Uses

Seeds can be sprouted and used in salads. Leaves may be eaten raw or cooked.

Caution

Do not take alfafa if you are suffering from an autoimmune condition such as systemic lupus elythematosus.

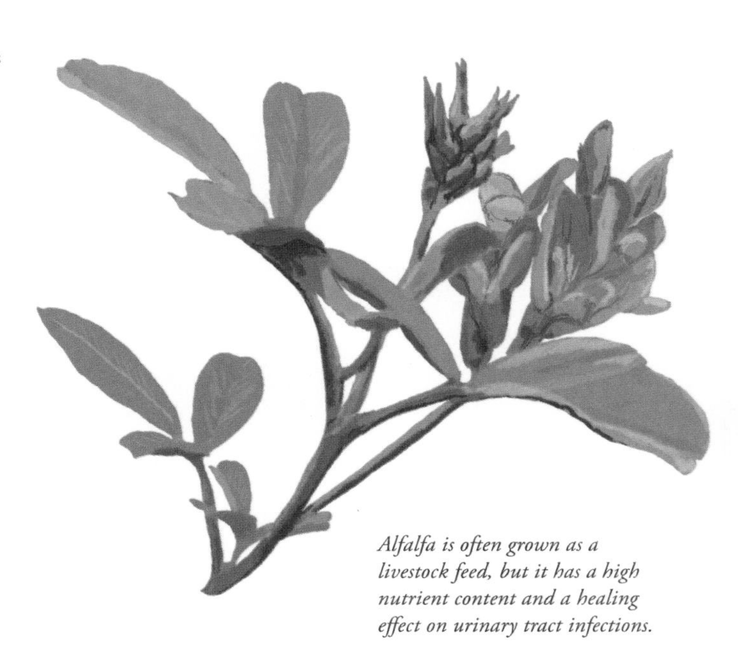

Alfalfa is often grown as a livestock feed, but it has a high nutrient content and a healing effect on urinary tract infections.

Lemon Balm
Melissa officinalis

This lemon-scented herb has powerful antiviral and antibacterial effects, which can be helpful in the treatment of recurrent cold sores. An application of a lemon balm-based cream just as the cold sore is forming can prevent it from erupting.

Origins & Characteristics
Taken internally, the herb helps with nervous problems and excitability, especially in children. Those who suffer from panic attacks and heart palpitations may find the extract helpful, as the herb has a sedative action and relaxes the nervous system.

For the treatment of depression, try an external application of lemon balm in an aromatherapy massage. Some people may prefer an all-over body massage, while others may prefer to have the upper back and shoulders massaged as an anti-stress technique.

Parts Used
Whole plant

Dosage
For external application, use as a cream. Apply enough to cover the area three times a day.

For aromatherapy application, use 6 drops of oil mixed with 2 teaspoons of almond oil. Massage in the usual way.

As a liquid tincture, take 15 drops twice daily.

Potential Benefits
- Has antiviral and antibacterial action
- Calms the nervous system
- Helps panic attacks
- Can help relieve depression

Cosmetic Uses
Used in cleansing lotions and as an infusion for relaxing baths.

Culinary Uses
Add the leaves to soups, salads and fish dishes. Lemon balm cordial can be purchased. It is similar to an elixir but is diluted with water before it is taken. It also forms a vital ingredient in the liqueur Benedictine.

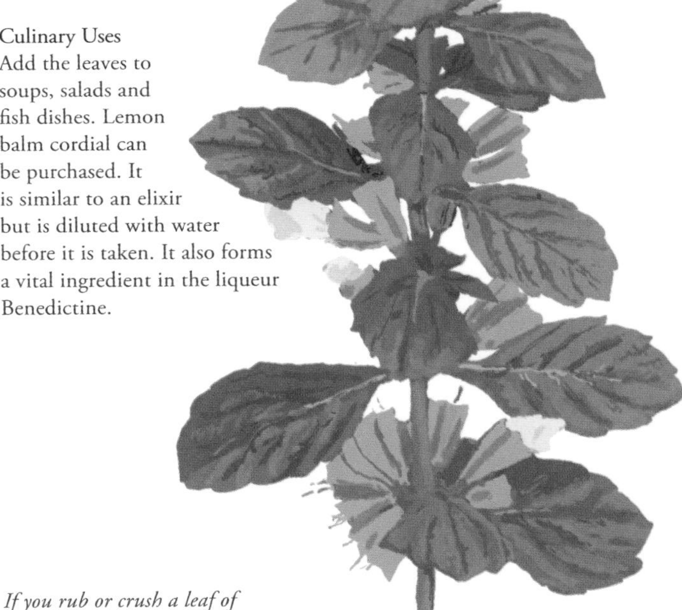

If you rub or crush a leaf of lemon balm it will release a distinct lemony aroma.

Peppermint
Mentha piperita

This strongly aromatic herb has a long history as a decongestant and antiseptic agent and is valuable in the treatment of colds and nasal congestion. The oils contained in the plant have a powerful antispasmodic action on the smooth muscle of the stomach, making it the herb of choice for adult colic, dyspepsia and irritable bowel syndrome.

Origins & Characteristics
The external application of the oil can help muscular discomfort and neuralgia. As a remedy for nausea and morning sickness, the normal internal dose of peppermint is very safe for a pregnant woman. Peppermint is also good for relieving menstrual pain as it has a relaxing effect.

Parts Used
Whole plant

Dosage
2 or 3 commercially prepared capsules (2ml of oil per capsule) taken between meals can relieve bowel spasms. As a tea, take 250ml (9fl oz) twice daily.

As an aromatherapy massage, use 6 drops of essential oil mixed with 2 teaspoons of almond oil.

Potential Benefits
- Has an antispasmodic agent for bowels
- Reduces nausea and sickness associated with early pregnancy
- Reduces stiffness when used as a muscle rub
- Has a decongestant action

Culinary Uses
Add the leaves to iced tea for a refreshing drink.

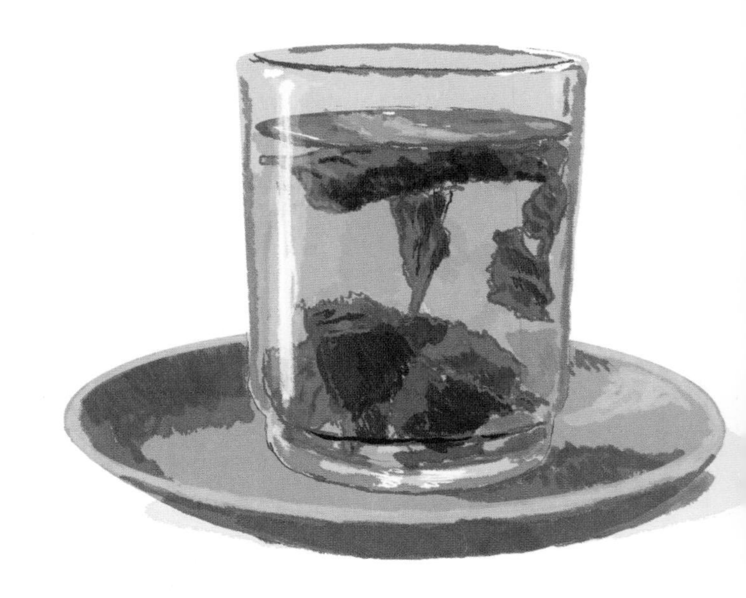

Peppermint tea makes a relaxing, caffeine-free drink at bedtime.

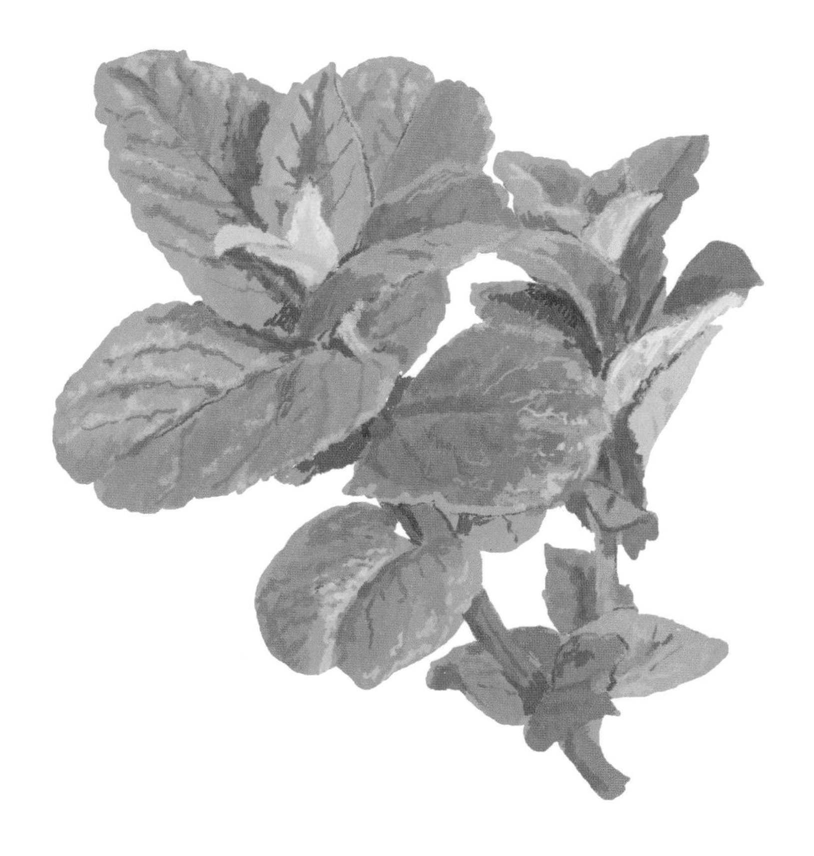

Peppermint is a popular remedy for digestive discomfort and nausea.

Basil
Ocimum basilicum

Basil is sometime referred to as St. Joseph's wort, not to be confused with St. John's wort. Its use dates back to biblical times, when it was seen after the resurrection growing around Christ's tomb. The word 'basil' is thought to come from the Greek for 'king'. Rich in volatile oils, basil contains over 20 chemical substances, including methyl cinnamate (cinnamon), citral (lemon), thymol (thyme), and camphor. There have been many variants of basil cultivated, each with a different aroma and flavour, making identification of different varieties difficult.

Origins & Characteristics
Basil has been taken internally for chills, colds and flu, in which it has a stimulant action. For digestion, basil is of great help in cases of stomach inflammation and helps relieve the abdominal cramps associated with menstruation.

Parts Used
Whole plant

Dosage
As a liquid tincture, take 15 drops twice daily.

Potential Benefits
- Acts as a stimulant and aids resistance to infection
- Soothes an inflamed stomach and aids digestion
- Has an antispasmodic action

Culinary Uses
Basil has many uses in cooking. The leaves make a good addition to any salad, adding a special flavour. Basil forms the basis of pesto, a traditional pasta sauce, as well as many stuffings for meat.

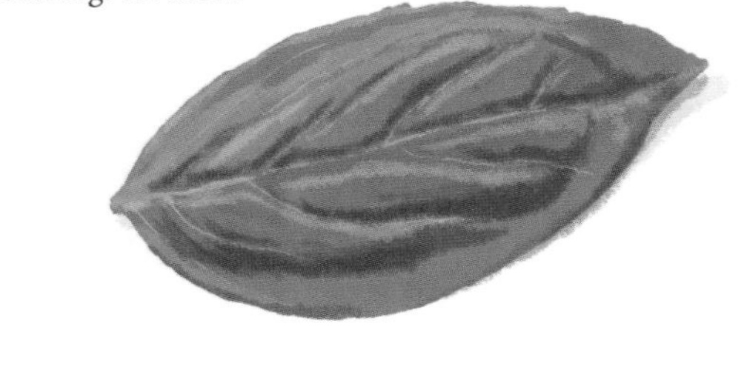

 CLASSIC BASIL PESTO

You will need:

- 2 garlic cloves
- 100g (4oz) fresh basil leaves
- 3 tbsp pinenuts
- sea salt
- 50g (2oz) Parmesan cheese, finely grated
- 8 tbsp extra virgin olive oil

Peel the garlic then crush in a mortar with the basil, pinenuts and a pinch of salt or blitz in a food processor. Once ground to a paste, mix in the oil and cheese. Store in a jar. Serve with pasta or spread on lightly toasted bread crostini.

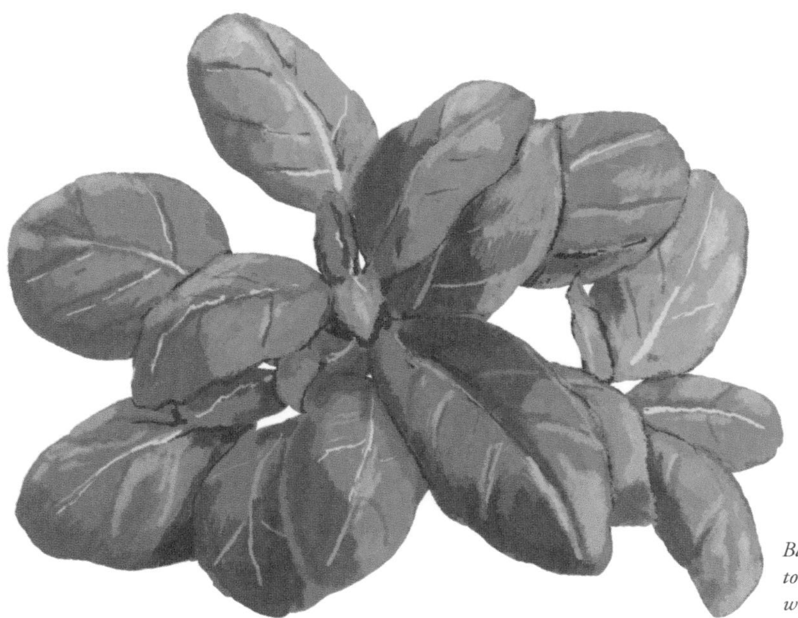

Basil is an easy herb to grow on a kitchen windowsill.

Evening Primrose
Oenothera biennis

This herb has risen to fame as a remedy for premenstrual and menopause symptoms, but there is a lot more to evening primrose than this. It is a very rich source of gamma linoleic acid (GLA), which is an essential fatty acid. GLA is vital for the health of cell membranes and balances the output of hormones. Taking evening primrose oil can block the action of these substances and reduce the discomfort. A dose of this oil can rebalance the hormonal system itself.

Origins & Characteristics
Gamma linoleic acid helps the body to produce prostaglandins, a hormone-like substance that helps to protect heart health. The positive effect of these prostaglandins may explain how evening primrose oil can appear to reduce blood pressure and the level of free cholesterol circulating in the blood.

As a remedy for skin problems, evening primrose is safe to use topically on a baby's cradle cap and, should eczema develop, evening primrose can be taken internally. Soap containing evening primrose oil is good for moisturising the skin.

It is interesting to note that schizophrenia has responded well to evening primrose supplements, although the mechanism behind this is unknown.

Parts Used
Oil

Dosage
For menopausal symptoms, take 2 or 3 capsules (500mg capsules) every evening with water only.

For premenstrual symptoms, take 3 capsules (500mg capsules) every evening for about 14 days before the onset of menstruation.

For children, use about 250mg of oil mixed in food daily.

For cradle cap, massage enough to make the area supple.

Potential Benefits
- Balances hormones
- Acts as an antispasmodic agent for abdominal cramps
- Lowers blood pressure
- Lowers cholesterol levels
- Helps eczema
- Helps schizophrenic symptoms

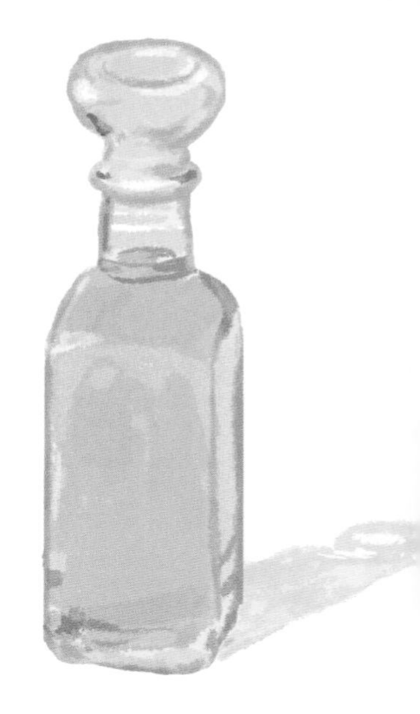

Evening primrose oil is usually taken as capsules, but the oil itself can be applied to dry skin or cradle cap.

Caution
Do not use if you suffer from epilepsy or migraines.

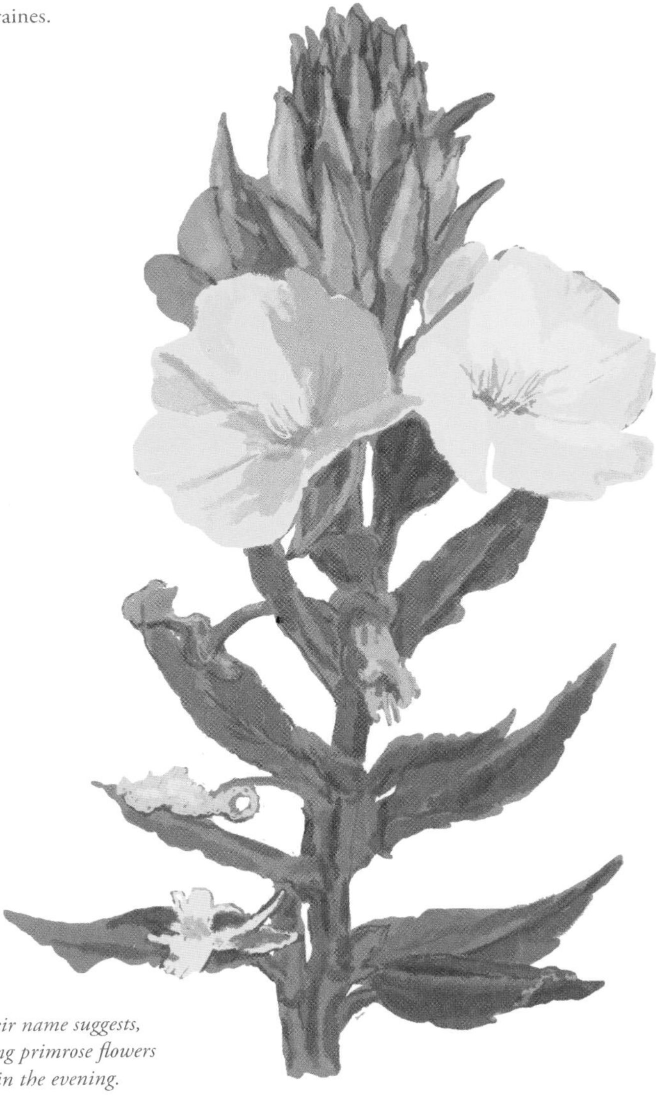

As their name suggests, evening primrose flowers open in the evening.

Olive
Olea europaea

The use of olive oil in cooking is well known, but for medicinal purposes, extracts are taken from the leaves as well as the fruits themselves. Leaf extracts can be used for the treatment of high blood pressure and nervous tension, while the oil extracted from the fruits aids in cases of constipation. The heart's health is greatly improved by the use of olive oil (best taken as the cold-pressed extra-virgin type) in cooking and food preparation.

Origins & Characteristics
Olive oil has the ability to reduce the bad cholesterol levels without affecting the beneficial cholesterol levels. Because olive oil is monounsaturated, there is little risk of free-radical generation if food is not cooked at very high temperatures.

Parts Used
Leaves and fruits

Dosage
As a laxative, take 2 or 3 tablespoons of oil.

For general health, use 1 or 2 tablespoons daily, mixed with food.

Potential Benefits
- Acts as a heart protector
- Reduces LDL cholesterol levels
- Reduces high blood pressure
- Acts to relax nerves and tension-related problems
- Helps relieve constipation

Culinary Uses
Use the oil for cooking as you would any other oil, but do not try to cook at very high temperatures. The oil can also be used instead of butter. Chop and use the fruits in pasta sauces and in bread mixes.

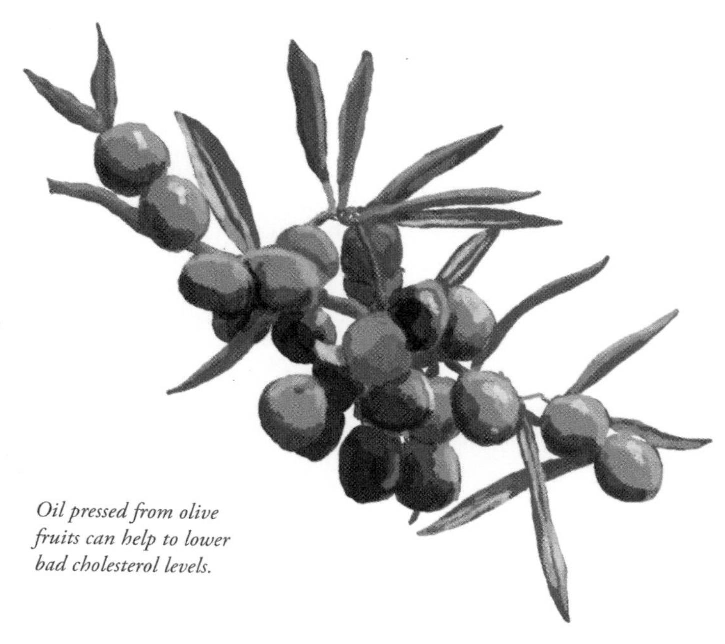

Oil pressed from olive fruits can help to lower bad cholesterol levels.

Sweet Marjoram

Origanum majorana

This is a popular culinary herb and is used in a variety of dishes. It is used to help digestion and reduce flatulence. Marjoram is a good antiseptic as it contains a large amount of thymol. It also has a very calming effect on the nerves and is helpful in relieving tension and menstrual cramps. It is helpful when the oil is massaged in an aromatherapy application.

Origins & Characteristics

Marjoram can be used to soothe sprains and many muscular aches and pains.

Apply a cold compress to sprains and a hot compress to aches and pains. Marjoram oil can also help with arthritis and rheumatism. Drinking a marjoram infusion can help fight colds and relieve bronchitis.

Marjoram can give temporary relief from toothache if the leaves are chewed.

Parts Used

Leaves and essential oil

Dosage

As an aromatherapy massage, use 6 drops of essential oil mixed with 2 teaspoons of almond oil. Massage the oils into the skin.

As a tea, infuse 2 teaspoons dried leaves in 250ml (9fl oz) of water and let stand for 5 minutes before drinking.

Potential Benefits

- Aids digestion
- Relieves tension
- Helps relieve menstrual cramps
- Fights colds
- Relieves arthritis and rheumatism
- Relieves toothache temporarily

Cosmetic Uses

Add an infusion of leaves for a relaxing bath.

Culinary Uses

Add leaves to casseroles, sauces and egg-and-cheese dishes.

Caution

Avoid during pregnancy.

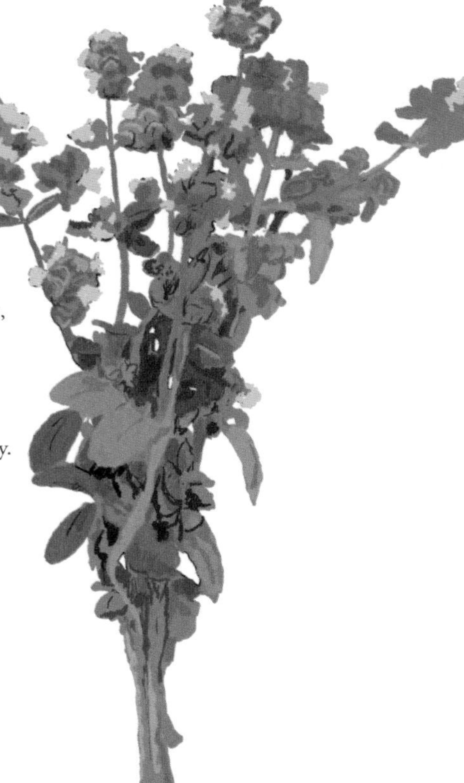

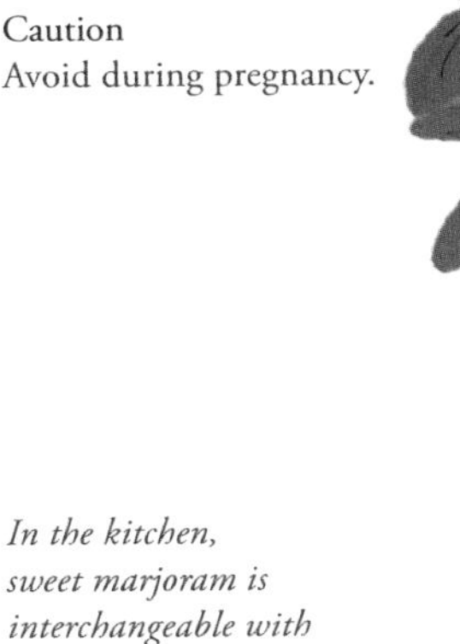

In the kitchen, sweet marjoram is interchangeable with oregano (Origanum vulgare).

Ginseng
Panax ginseng

Panax is derived from the word panacea, meaning a treatment for all problems. The Chinese, some 5,000 years ago, attributed to ginseng many properties and cures. When taken internally, ginseng acts as a general tonic by stimulating the central nervous system.

Origins & Characteristics

Ginseng has been shown to reduce the blood concentrations of both glucose and cholesterol as well as stimulating resistance to disease. It also has a reputation for being an aphrodisiac.

Ginseng encourages the secretion of hormones to improve stamina and may be used to treat stress and chronic fatigue.

Parts Used

Root

Dosage

Take 2 teaspoons of ginseng elixir daily for up to two weeks.

Potential Benefits

- Stimulates the central nervous system
- Improves stamina
- Boosts resistance to infection
- Reduces blood glucose and cholesterol levels
- May act as an aphrodisiac

Caution

Ginseng should not be used continuously for more than one month. It may cause headaches.

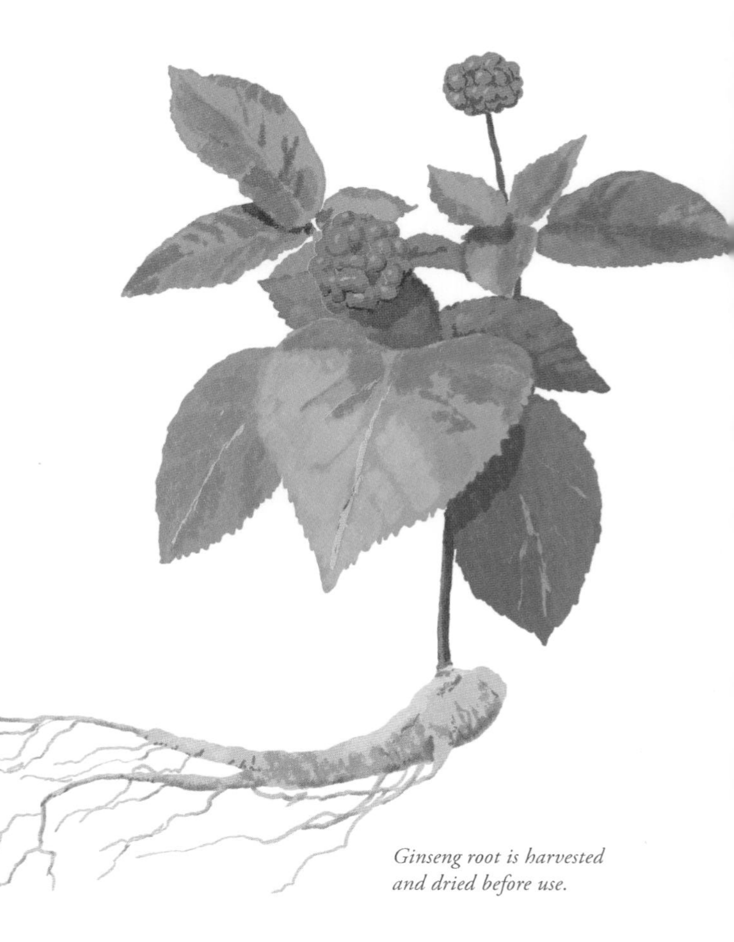

Ginseng root is harvested and dried before use.

Parsley
Petroselinum crispum

Parsley was first recorded in an early Greek herbal as long ago as the third century B.C. It was used in ancient Rome in cooking and in ceremonies. It is rich in vitamins A and C and contains flavonoids that help to reduce allergic reactions, but its main action appears to be detoxification.

Origins & Characteristics

An internal dose of parsley can help stimulate the menstrual process and help relieve menstrual cramps. The stimulant effect on the uterus makes this herb one to avoid during pregnancy, but once the baby is born, it may help stimulate lactation and milk flow.

Parsley also acts as an effective diuretic and helps relieve kidney complaints. It also helps reduce inflammation of the bladder as well as the prostate. In the stomach, it can help relieve colic, flatulence and indigestion.

Parts Used

Seeds, leaves, roots and oil extract

Dosage

As a liquid tincture, take 20 drops twice daily.

Potential Benefits

- Stimulates flow of breast milk
- Aids menstrual cramps
- Reduces inflammation in the bladder (cystitis)
- Stimulates the flow of urine
- Helps reduce colic and indigestion

Culinary Uses

Use in sauces and as a garnish for fish, cheese and egg dishes. Parsley can also be added to dressings and vinaigrettes.

Caution

Avoid during pregnancy.

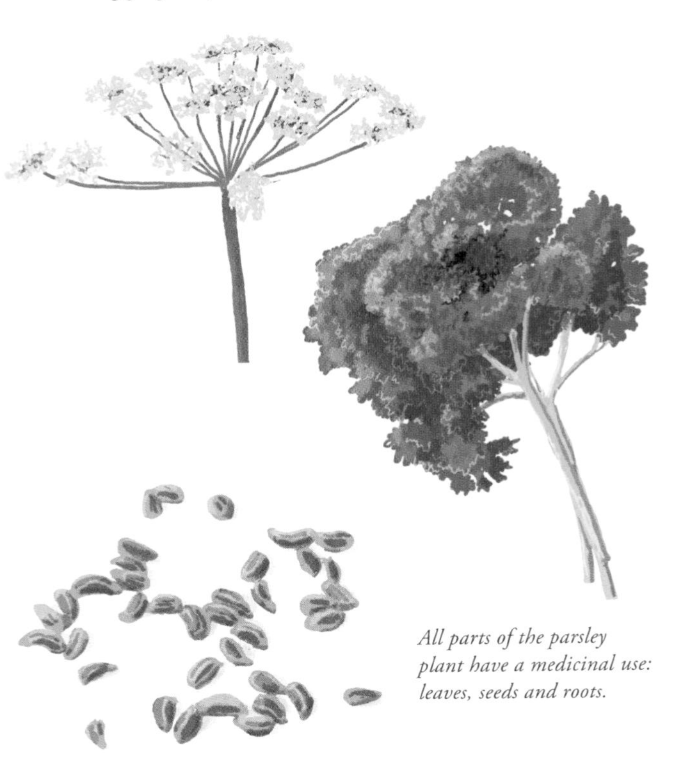

All parts of the parsley plant have a medicinal use: leaves, seeds and roots.

Kava Kava
Piper methysticum

This intoxicating pepper was made into a special drink by the Polynesians and given to Captain Cook. The resulting effects led him to name it botanically as 'intoxicating pepper'. Kava kava is still made into a drink by the Melanesians during certain rituals, when it is said to enhance mental awareness.

Origins & Characteristics
Herbalists today use this herb to stimulate the nervous and circulatory systems. It cures insomnia and nervousness by enhancing restfulness. Kava kava has the ability to reduce the pain associated with muscle spasms and arthritis.

Parts Used
Roots and rhizomes

Dosage
Take 2 tablets (100mg) of dried herb daily.

Potential Benefits
- Acts as a remedy for insomnia
- Acts as a nerve tonic
- Acts as a mental stimulant
- Reduces muscle spasms
- Helps reduce joint pains associated with rheumatism

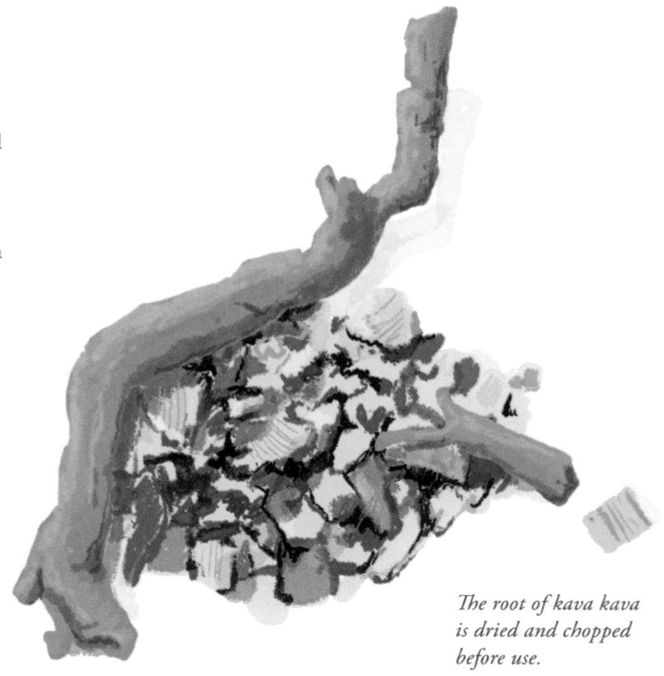

The root of kava kava is dried and chopped before use.

Greater Plantain
Plantago major

First discovered in ancient China in about 206 B.C., plantain was a popular medicine of the day. Its astringent properties promote healing and act as an effective expectorant in cases of chest infections. These properties led the herb to be used for cases of diarrhoea and bowel inflammation.

Origins & Characteristics
Externally, use the juice for ear infections, wounds, eye inflammation and haemorrhoids.

Parts Used
Leaves

Dosage
As a liquid tincture, take 20 drops twice daily. For external application, crush the leaves and collect the juice, then apply directly to the affected area.

Potential Benefits
- Cleanses wounds
- Has an antiseptic action
- Helps control diarrhoea and bowel inflammation
- Reduces ear and eye inflammation

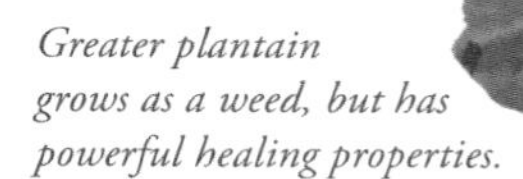

Greater plantain grows as a weed, but has powerful healing properties.

Tormentil or Bloodroot
Potentilla tormentilla

This rather unassuming plant has very thick and strong roots that, when cut, reveal a blood-red colour – hence the common name of bloodroot. Tormentil contains a high concentration of astringents, making it an important medicinal plant.

Origins & Characteristics
The action of this herb is mainly due to tannic acid, which makes it a useful preparation for treating diarrhoea and inflammatory problems affecting the mucous membranes of the mouth, throat and stomach. Externally, it can be used to help heal wounds and cuts.

Parts Used
Roots (rhizome)

Dosage
As a liquid tincture, take 2 drops twice daily after eating.
For external application, use as a poultice for wounds.

Potential Benefits
- Helps treat colitis
- Reduces diarrhoea
- Soothes an irritated throat
- Reduces inflammation of the lining of the mouth
- Helps heal wounds and cuts

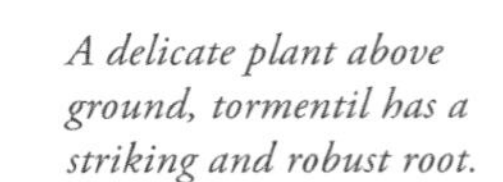

A delicate plant above ground, tormentil has a striking and robust root.

Blackthorn
Prunus spinosa

Blackthorn contains very powerful chemicals (anthraquinone glycosides) that stimulate the contraction of the bowel wall, causing nausea, abdominal cramping and vomiting. Storing the herb for a number of years will reduce this effect.

Origins & Characteristics
Because of its action in causing nausea, blackthorn has been used as a purgative (to induce vomiting) and, in smaller doses, as a laxative.

Parts Used
Bark and fruits

Dosage
As a liquid tincture, take 20 drops daily.

Potential Benefits
- Acts as a very effective laxative
- Acts as a purgative
- Acts as a diuretic

Caution
This herb is very strong. Over-dosage will cause vomiting and diarrhoea.

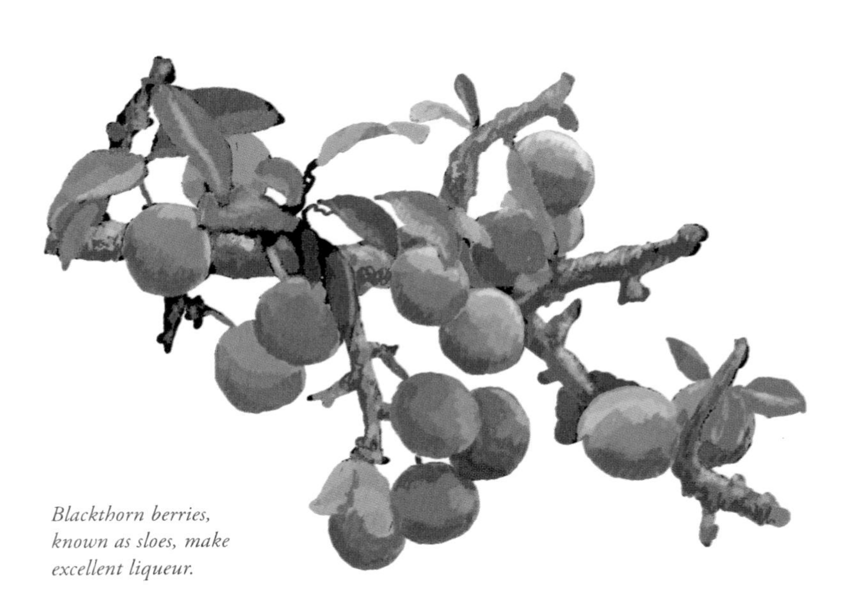

Blackthorn berries, known as sloes, make excellent liqueur.

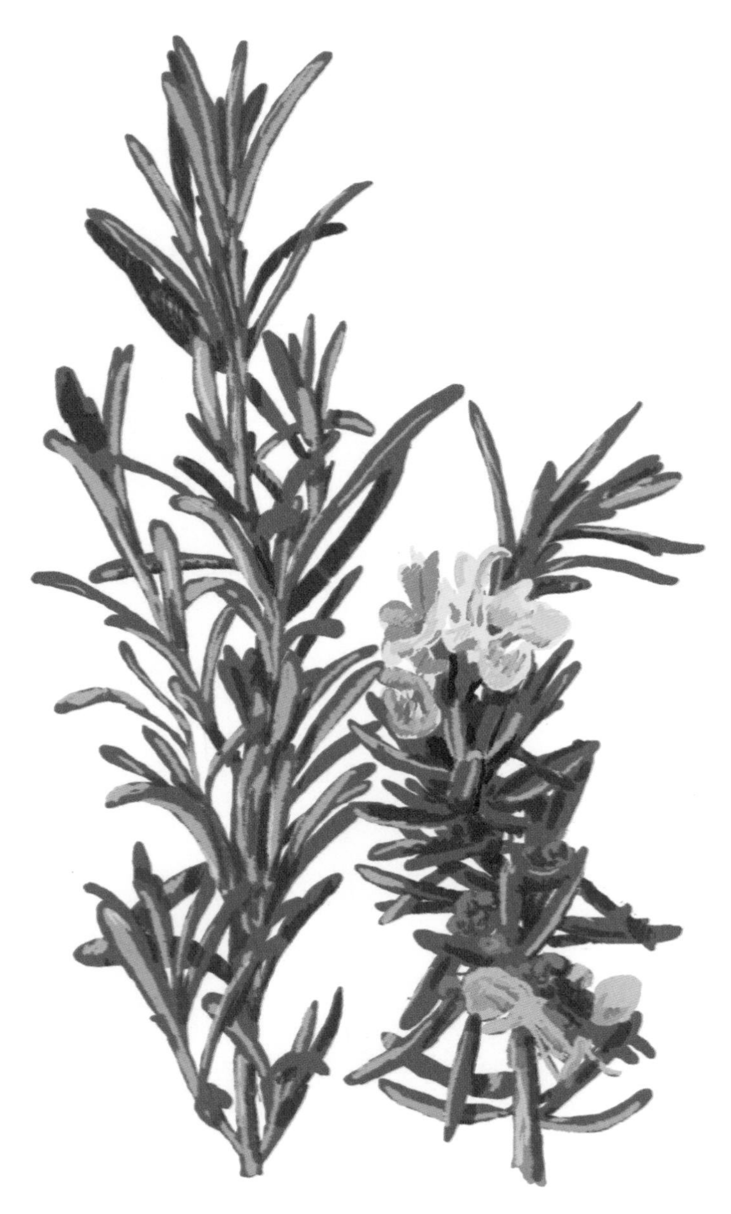

Rosemary grows into a large, bushy shrub. Its aromatic, needle-like leaves are evergreen, but it flowers in summer.

Rosemary
Rosmarinus officinalis

Rich in volatile oils, rosemary is a very strong antiseptic agent with powerful anti-inflammatory actions. The phenolic acid content of rosemary is responsible for this anti-microbial property and it has been used as an effective anti-infective agent for many hundreds of years.

Origins & Characteristics

In addition to its anti-inflammatory and anti-microbial properties, the internal use of rosemary includes the treatment of depression, fatigue, migraine and tension headaches, poor circulation, and digestive disorders, including flatulence. Rosemary acts as a good circulatory stimulant and has a balancing and calming effect on the digestive system.

For rheumatism and muscular aches, the external application of rosemary oil can give relief. The oil can also be used as an insect repellent and the dried leaves can be used in potpourri and to scent clothes and linen.

Traditionally, an infusion of rosemary has been used as a shampoo to stimulate hair growth and as a rinse to lighten blonde hair.

Parts Used

Leaves, flowering tips and essential oil

Dosage

As an external application, apply 6 drops of essential oil, mixed with 2 teaspoons of almond oil, to the desired area twice daily. As a liquid tincture, take 10 drops twice daily.

As a tea, add a teaspoon of chopped leaves to 250ml (9fl oz) of boiling water and let stand for 5 minutes.

Potential Benefits

- Acts as all antiseptic agent for cuts and wounds
- Has an anti-depressant activity
- Reduces headache and migraine symptoms
- Stimulates circulation and digestion
- Relieves flatulence

Culinary Uses

Rosemary is especially good with lamb and in soups and stews. Leave a fresh sprig in oil to steep for 1 month to produce a flavoured oil, that must be refrigerated and used quickly.

Caution

The essential oil should not be used internally.

Raspberry Leaves
Rubus idaeus

Raspberries have formed part of the human diet for as long as fossil records date back; they were even mentioned in the writings of Hippocrates (460–370 B.C.). As a remedy for menstrual cramps, raspberry tea appears to be very effective.

Origins & Characteristics

The astringent properties of this herb can be of use to pregnant women to tone up the uterine muscles. It is often given in preparation for childbirth and also for a couple of months after birth to help restore the tone of the uterus.

Parts Used

Leaves and fruits

Dosage

As a tea, add a teaspoon of raspberry leaves (or use a commercial preparation) to 250ml (9fl oz) of boiling water and drink twice daily during the third trimester of pregnancy.

As a remedy for menstrual cramps, sip the tea as needed.

Potential Benefits

- Aids labour in childbirth
- Tones up the uterus
- Reduces menstrual cramps

Caution

The use of this herb during pregnancy should be restricted to the third trimester.

The fruit of the raspberry takes all the glory, but don't overlook the leaves.

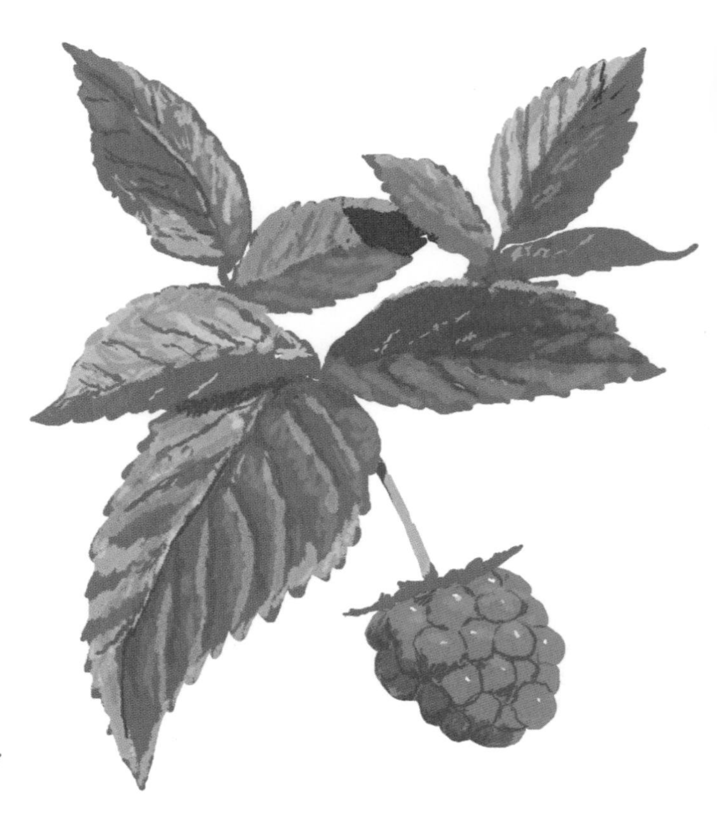

Butcher's Broom
Ruscus aculeatus

As far back as the first century A.D., butcher's broom was known to have medicinal properties, and it was mentioned as a treatment for kidney stones. Modern techniques have now identified the active agent, a steroid-like substance that can effectively reduce inflammation by constricting the veins.

Origins & Characteristics
A popular use for this herb is as a mild diuretic. When butcher's broom is taken internally, the circulatory system benefits from its tonic action, and improvements in poor circulation and in cases of haemorrhoids have been reported.

An external application can be soothing when applied to painful haemorrhoids.

Parts Used
Young shoots and roots

Dosage
As a liquid tincture, take 15 drops twice daily.

For external application, use as a cream, as required.

Potential Benefits
- Acts as a circulatory tonic
- Has an anti-inflammatory action
- Acts as a mild diuretic to reduce swollen ankles
- Helps relieve the pain of arthritis

Caution
Avoid in cases of high blood pressure.

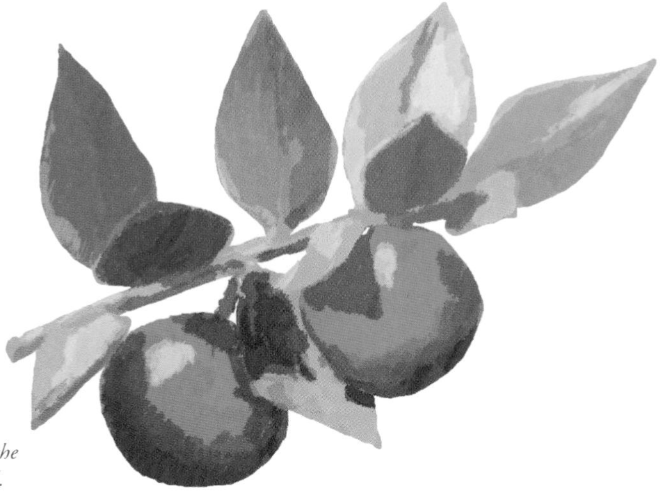

Butcher's broom's scarlet berries do not have medicinal properties; the young shoots and the roots are used.

White Willow
Salix alba

Salix contains a natural aspirin-like substance, salicylic acid, which was first produced commercially in 1838. Like aspirin, white willow's healing actions include the reduction of fever, improvement in joint stiffness associated with arthritis and rheumatism, symptomatic easing of headaches and reduction of inflammation.

Origins & Characteristics

It is interesting to note that pure salicylic acid intake is associated with stomach irritation, but that its presence in the white willow is buffered by tannins, which actually protect the stomach.

Parts Used

Leaves and bark

Dosage

As a liquid tincture, take 20 drops twice daily after eating.

Potential Benefits

- Acts as an anti-inflammatory agent
- Helps treat arthritis and rheumatism
- Reduces fevers

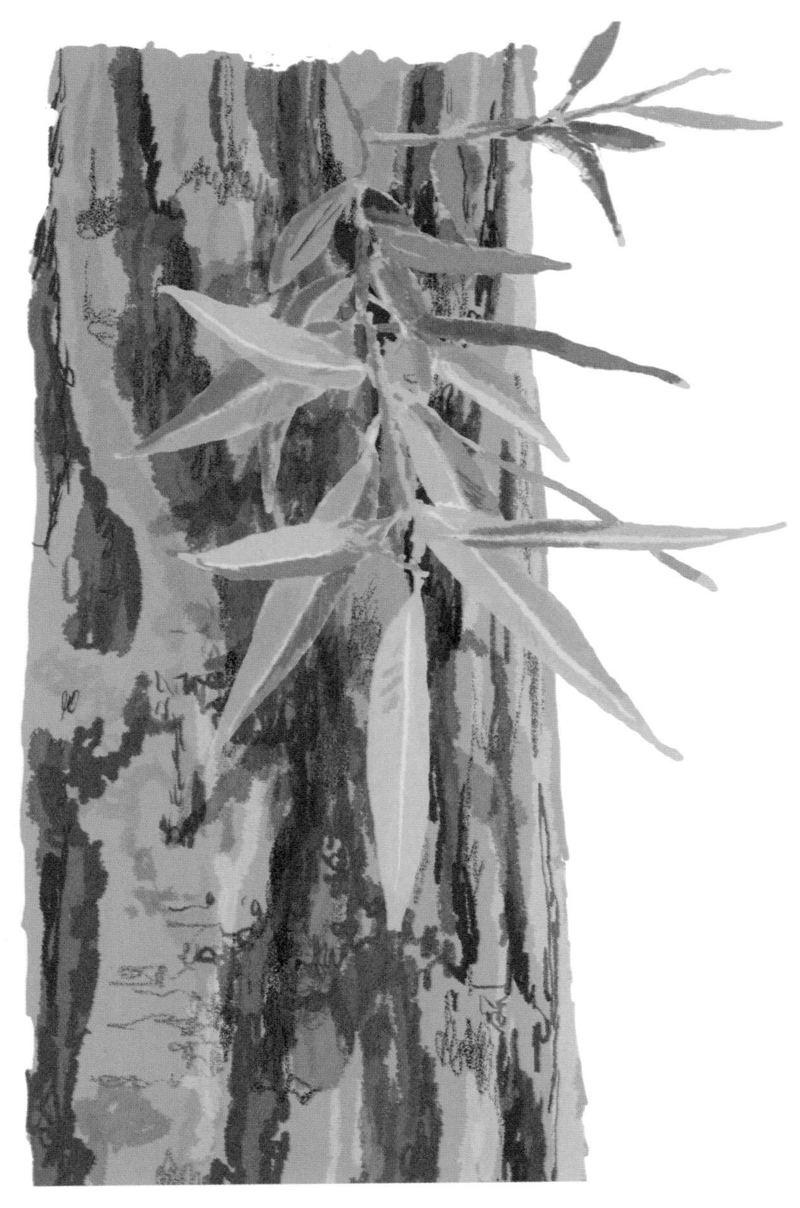

You may find relief from aches and pains by chewing pieces of white willow bark, but powder and liquid forms are also available.

Sage
Salvia officinalis

Sage was associated with long life in the eighteenth century and was a cherished herb. A wide array of aromas can be noticed coming from freshly cut sage due to the high content of volatile oils present in the plant. Sage provides us with a readily available antiseptic agent. Fresh sage juice has anti-inflammatory and antiseptic activities. It can be used as a mouthwash and a gargle for tonsillitis and laryngitis. Sage can be used externally in a compress to promote the healing of wounds.

Origins & Characteristics

Sage extracts can effectively relax smooth muscles (found in the internal organs), and it has an effect on the female chemistry rather like that of oestrogen. This oestrogenic effect can actually reduce and suppress the production of breast milk. Sage can, therefore, be taken to control excessive lactation. The oestrogen-like stimulation of sage can help relieve menopausal problems, and sage has been used to assist fertility.

People with indigestion and digestive problems such as dyspepsia benefit from this herb and, taken as a tea, sage is useful for combatting stress.

There are more than 750 different species in the sage family. One, *Salvia sclarea*, or 'clary sage' (also known as muscatel) is derived from the folkloric words 'clear eye'. The volatile oil from this sage is used in aromatherapy massage and has many therapeutic actions. It is very effective as an anti-depressant. It has a calming effect and can act as a sedative. Clary is also used as a general tonic for the whole body and helps to relieve menstrual cramps. This oil blends very well with sandalwood (*Santalum album*) and lavender (*Lavandula officinalis*), and it is safe to use on children.

Parts Used

Leaves

Dosage

As a liquid tincture, take 20 drops twice daily.

For external application, use as a compress for wounds.

As a clary sage aromatherapy application, use 3 drops in 1 teaspoon of almond oil and massage in the usual way.

As a clary sage bath for children, add 2 drops in 1 teaspoon of almond oil and mix in the bath.

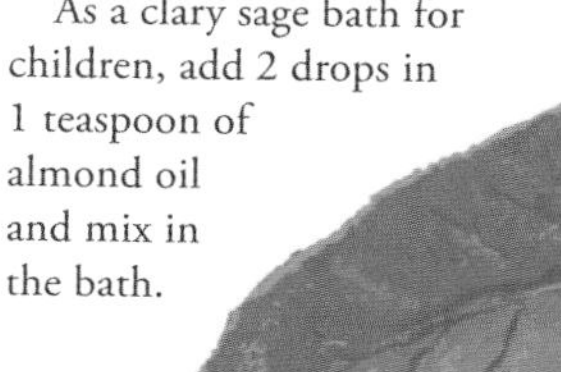

Potential Benefits

- Stimulates fertility
- Helps relieve menopausal problems
- Reduces excessive milk production in lactating women
- Has antiseptic and anti-inflammatory effects

Clary sage

- Relieves depression
- Has a calming effect
- Helps reduce menstrual cramps

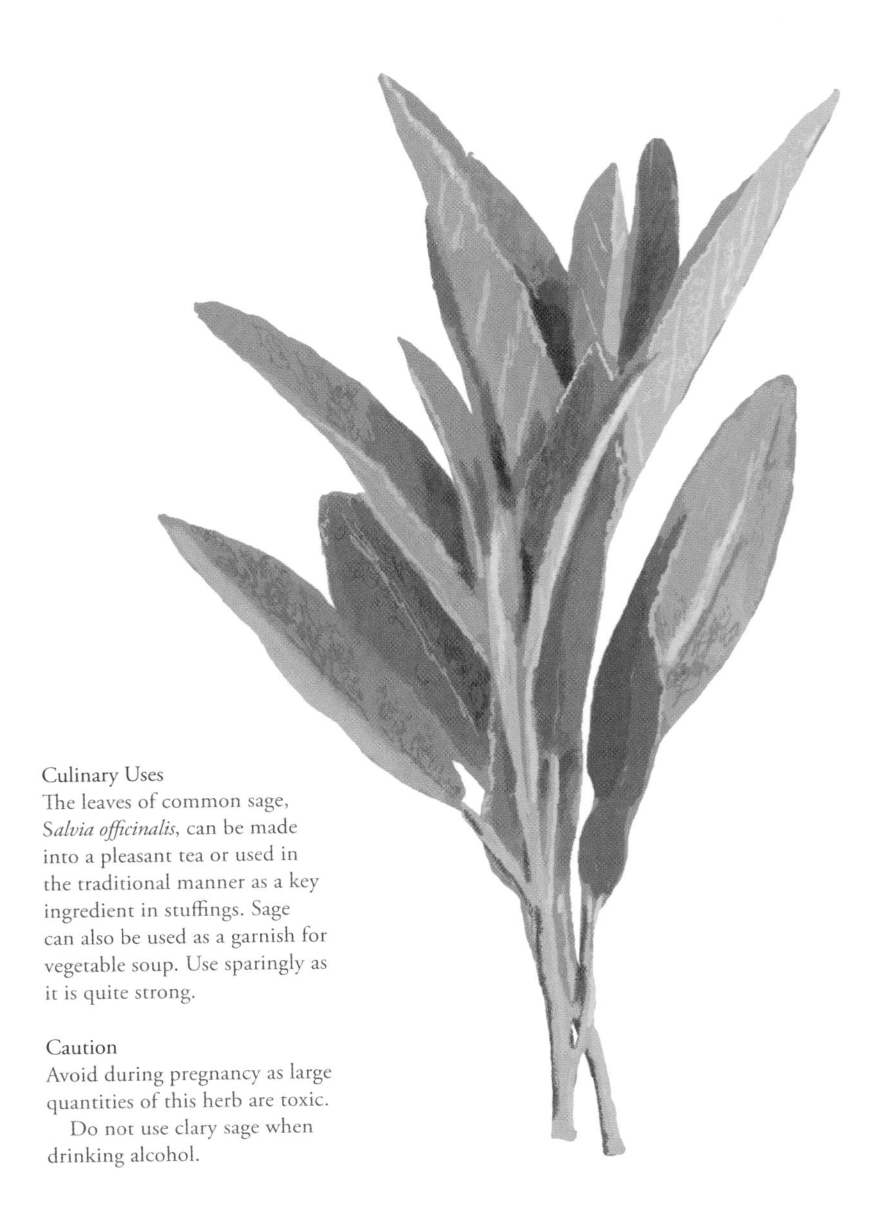

Culinary Uses
The leaves of common sage, *Salvia officinalis*, can be made into a pleasant tea or used in the traditional manner as a key ingredient in stuffings. Sage can also be used as a garnish for vegetable soup. Use sparingly as it is quite strong.

Caution
Avoid during pregnancy as large quantities of this herb are toxic.
Do not use clary sage when drinking alcohol.

Common sage has soft green leaves, but other varieties may be variegated or even purple.

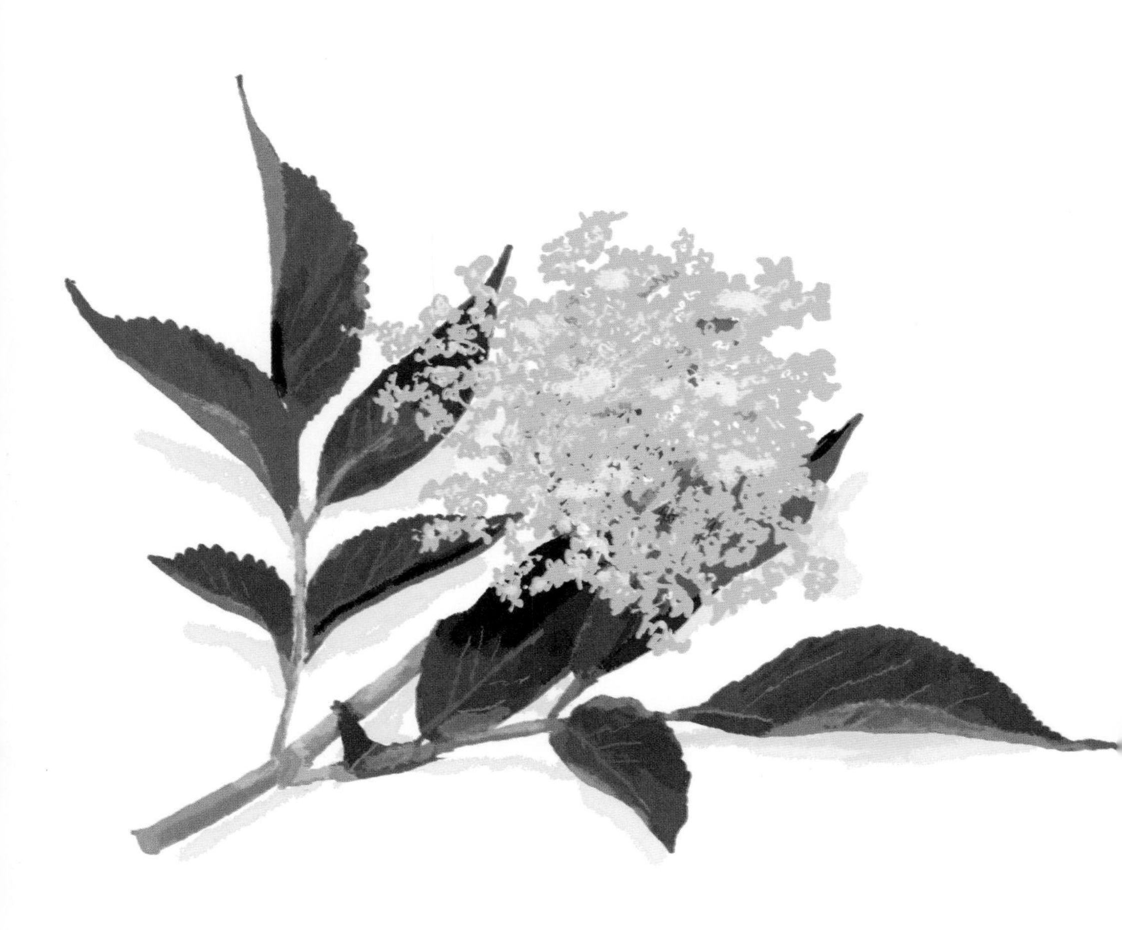

Fragrant elderflowers make a delicious summer cordial or a tonic to tone and lighten the skin.

Elder
Sambucus nigra

When a cold is on its way, drink a hot tea made from elder. This will stimulate an increase in body temperature, which will help your body to speed the killing of the invading bacteria or virus.

Origins & Characteristics
Elder has very effective decongestant properties and can be combined with many herbs to boost their activity in combatting chest infections, nasal congestion and chills. This herb can also help relieve hay fever, bronchial congestion and sinusitis.

The fruits of the elder tree can be used in relieving rheumatic joint problems. An external application of elder can be of great relief to irritated skin, bruises, sprains and minor wounds. It can be applied to the skin as an infusion or ointment.

Elderflower water can be used as an effective skin toner, lightener and to fade away any unwanted freckles.

Parts Used
Leaves, bark, flowers and fruits

Dosage
A remedy made from elderberry juice boiled with sugar to make a syrup is good taken twice daily for bronchitis and colds.

For external application, use as a cream as required.

Potential Benefits
- Helps clear colds and flu
- Increases body temperature to assist in the elimination of invading infections
- Helps relieve sinusitis
- Soothes irritated skin

Cosmetic Uses
Can be made into a cleansing milk and lotion to soften the skin.

Culinary Uses
Boil the juice from the fruits with a little sugar, ginger and a few cloves to produce elderberry rod (cordial).

Preserves and sauces can be made from the fruits.

Caution
The seeds from the elder can be toxic and should be avoided. Always cook the fruits first before eating them.

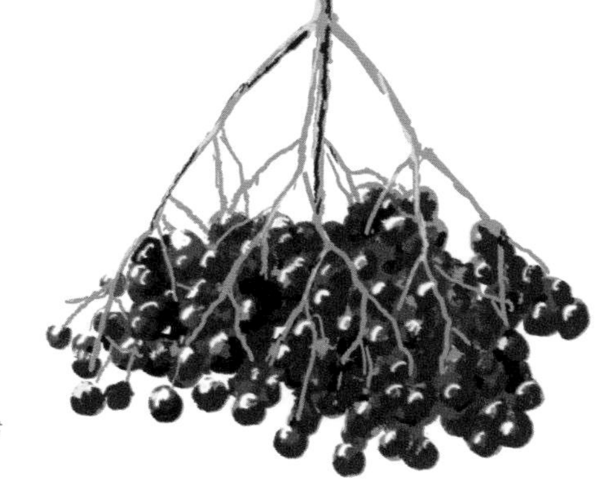

Elderberries make a good syrup to treat bronchitis.

Skullcap
Scutellaria baicalensis

First mentioned in Chinese writings dating back to A.D. 25–220, skullcap has been used in medicinal preparations ever since. Do not confuse it with American Skullcap (*Scutellaria lateriflora*), which is used to treat insomnia and anxiety and is a different variety.

Origins & Characteristics
Skullcap's active agents, such as certain flavonoids that improve liver function, make it an important remedy for all kinds of liver disease.

Its anti-inflammatory action also makes skullcap an effective treatment for poisonous bites, diarrhoea and pharyngitis.

American Skullcap is used to treat anxiety, depression and insomnia as it relaxes the nervous system. The plant was used by the Cherokee, to induce menstruation, but this use has now dwindled.

Parts Used
Roots

Dosage
As a liquid tincture, take 20 drops twice daily after eating.

Potential Benefits
- Can be used to treat liver disease
- Reduces inflammation of stomach and bowel
- Reduces diarrhoea
- Helps cases of sore throat
- Can help insomnia

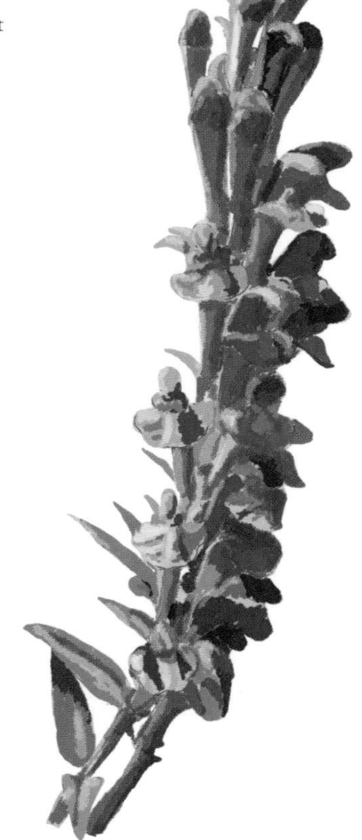

The roots of skullcap are dried before use. The purplish-blue flower spikes grow to 1.2m (4ft) tall.

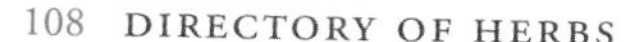

Milk Thistle
Silybum marianum

This powerful herb can counteract the damage of a lethal dose of the death cap mushroom (*Amanita phalloides*) and is particularly useful in counteracting liver complaints. It can even help to promote the regeneration of damaged liver cells.

Origins & Characteristics
Liver enzyme systems are protected by the silymarin content of this bitter herb. Liver function is not only protected by silymarin, but its function also appears to be enhanced and new liver cells can be seen to appear. This action is used to treat liver cirrhosis and hepatitis, both potentially fatal conditions.

Parts Used
Whole plant

Dosage
As a liquid tincture, take 20 drops twice daily.

Potential Benefits
- Acts as a powerful liver protector
- Helps fight hepatitis
- May help regenerate damaged liver cells

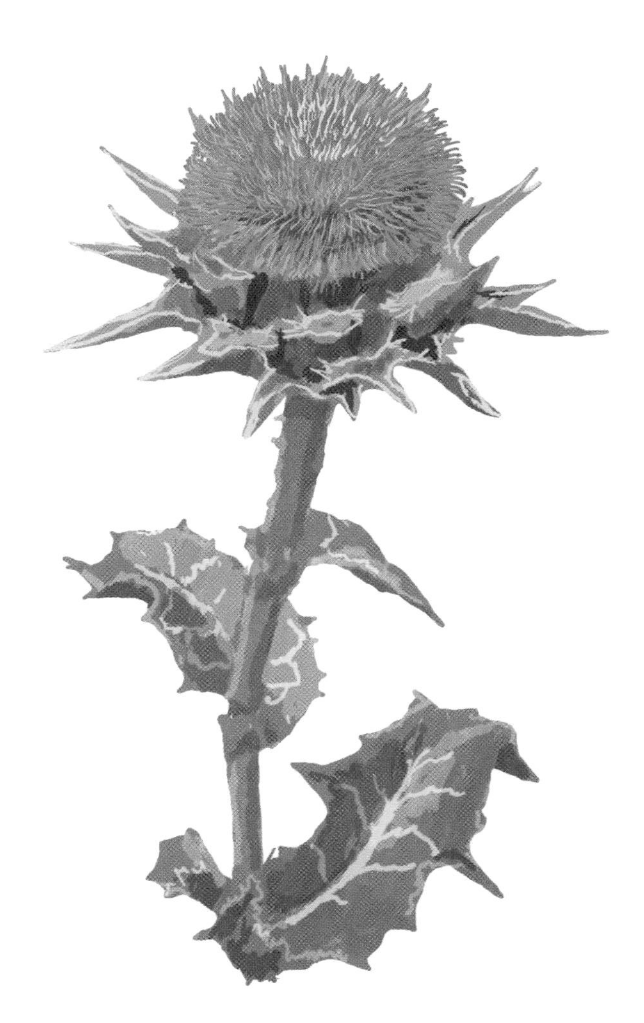

Milk thistle gets its common name from the milky liquid that comes from the leaves when they are crushed.

Comfrey
Symphytum officinale

Comfrey is probably one of the best-known medicinal herbs. Its use by herbalists can be traced back over many centuries and is related to borage (*Borago officinalis*). Comfrey is known under other names including knitbone as it can heal bone fractures.

Origins & Characteristics

Recent research work has isolated an active agent, a pyrrolizidine alkaloid, which is responsible for the healing actions of comfrey, but this substance can induce liver damage and tumours. For this reason, internal usage is not recommended.

Used externally, comfrey can speed the healing of wounds. Comfrey creams are perfectly safe and are very effective remedies for poorly healing wounds, eczema, psoriasis, haemorrhoids and skin ulcers.

A comfrey poultice can be used to help heal sprains and severe cuts and to soothe pain and inflammation. It can also be used to drain boils and abscesses.

Traditionally, comfrey cream has been used for the treatment of mastitis in nursing women, but, because of its possible toxic effects when taken internally, this should be avoided in case the infant should ingest some of the cream during feeding.

Parts Used

Leaves and roots

Dosage

For external application, use as a cream locally as required.

For external application use as a poultice as required.

Potential Benefits

- Heals skin
- Speeds the healing of wounds
- Soothes haemorrhoids
- Reduces inflammation associated with eczema and psoriasis
- Helps drain boils and abcesses
- Helps relieve sprains

Cosmetic Uses

Add an infusion of comfrey leaves for a healing bath.

May be used in a lotion to soften the skin.

Can be used in lip balm to protect the lips.

Caution

Do not take internally or use for the treatment of mastitis if breastfeeding.

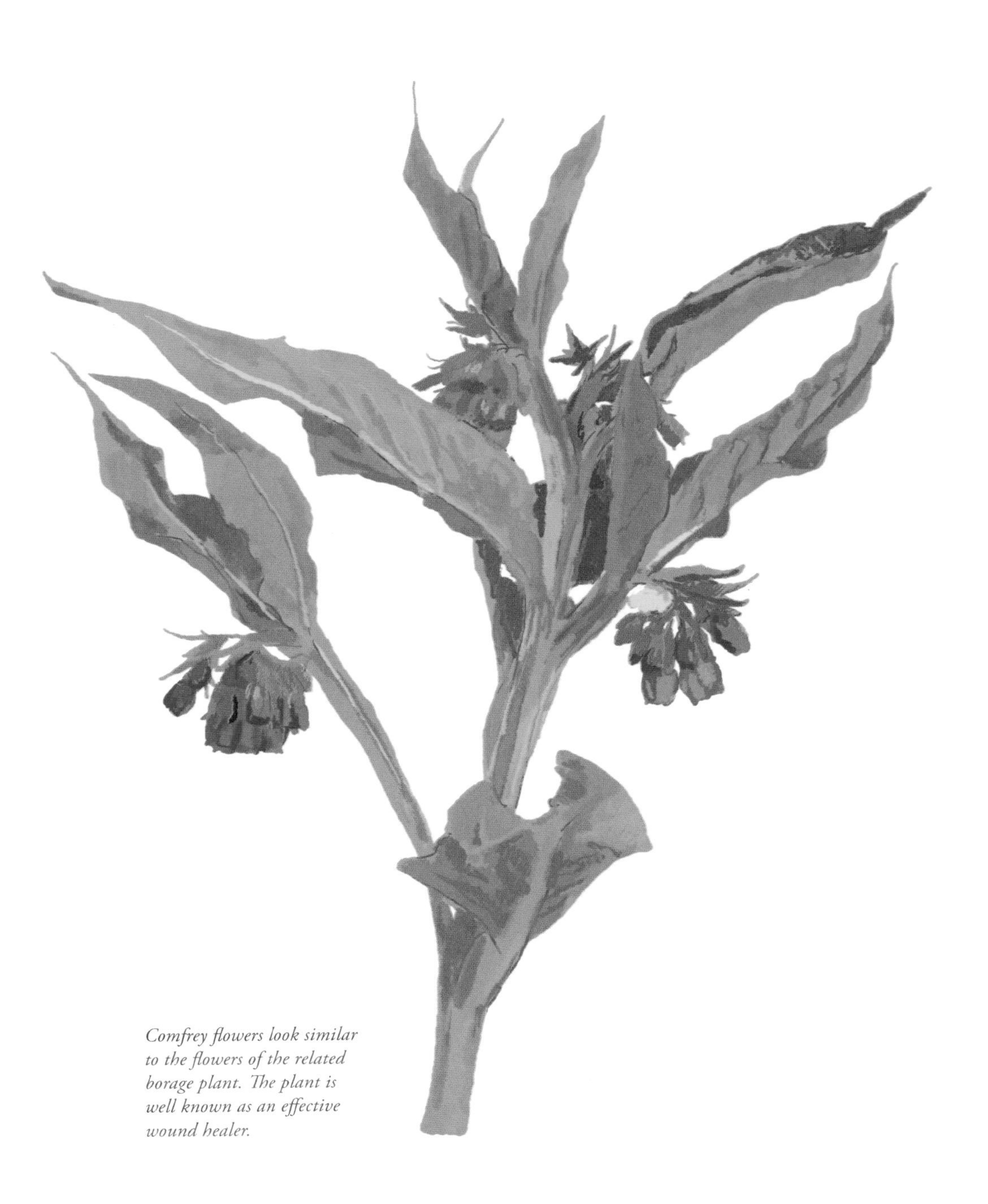

Comfrey flowers look similar to the flowers of the related borage plant. The plant is well known as an effective wound healer.

Cloves
Syzygium aromaticum

Fresh cloves look quite different from the dark twiglike dried herb we are used to seeing. As far back as A.D. 600, the Chinese were documented to use cloves for many different reasons. The volatile oil contained in cloves – eugenol – gives them their unique aroma. Another active constituent of cloves, methyl salicylate, has been recently identified and may be involved in the painkilling aspects attributed to clove extracts.

Origins & Characteristics
For toothache, clove oil should be used. Apply a small amount either directly on the tooth or use a cotton swab for difficult-to-reach areas. It is not recommended to leave absorbent cotton soaked in clove oil for too long in one place because the surrounding tissue of the mouth may suffer. When taken internally, cloves can help to settle an upset stomach, and ease the symptoms of nausea, chills and even impotence.

Parts Used
Flower buds and oil

Dosage
Apply a few drops of oil to a toothache 2 or 3 times a day.
Add 6 cloves to an herbal tea and let stand for 5 minutes.

Potential Benefits
- Helps an upset stomach
- Relieves chills and colds
- Acts as a toothache remedy

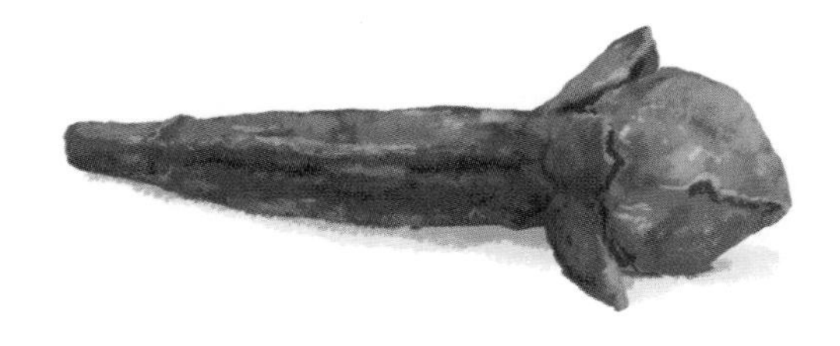

Each individual clove has a distinctive nail-like shape.

Culinary Uses

Cloves give a special flavour to preserved meats, especially ham. Stud a ham with cloves and wrap well. After a few days the ham will take on a hint of the clove flavour. Whole cloves can be added to an oil base and allowed to steep for a month to produce a flavoured cooking oil that should be refrigerated and used shortly. Cloves may also be used in pickling and baking.

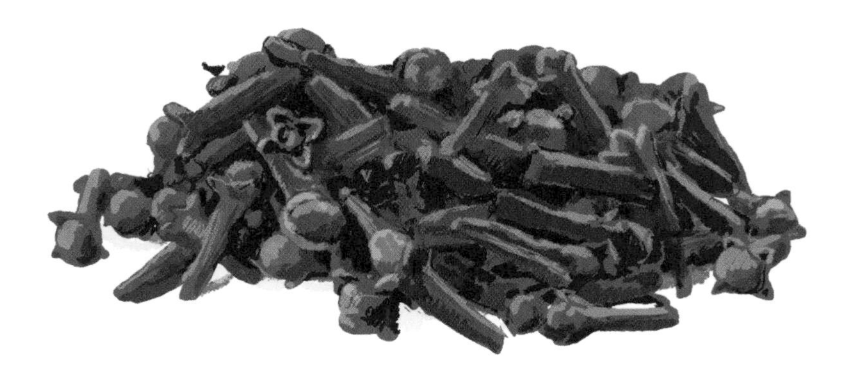

Cloves have an evocative aroma that conjures up images of the spice islands of the Indian Ocean.

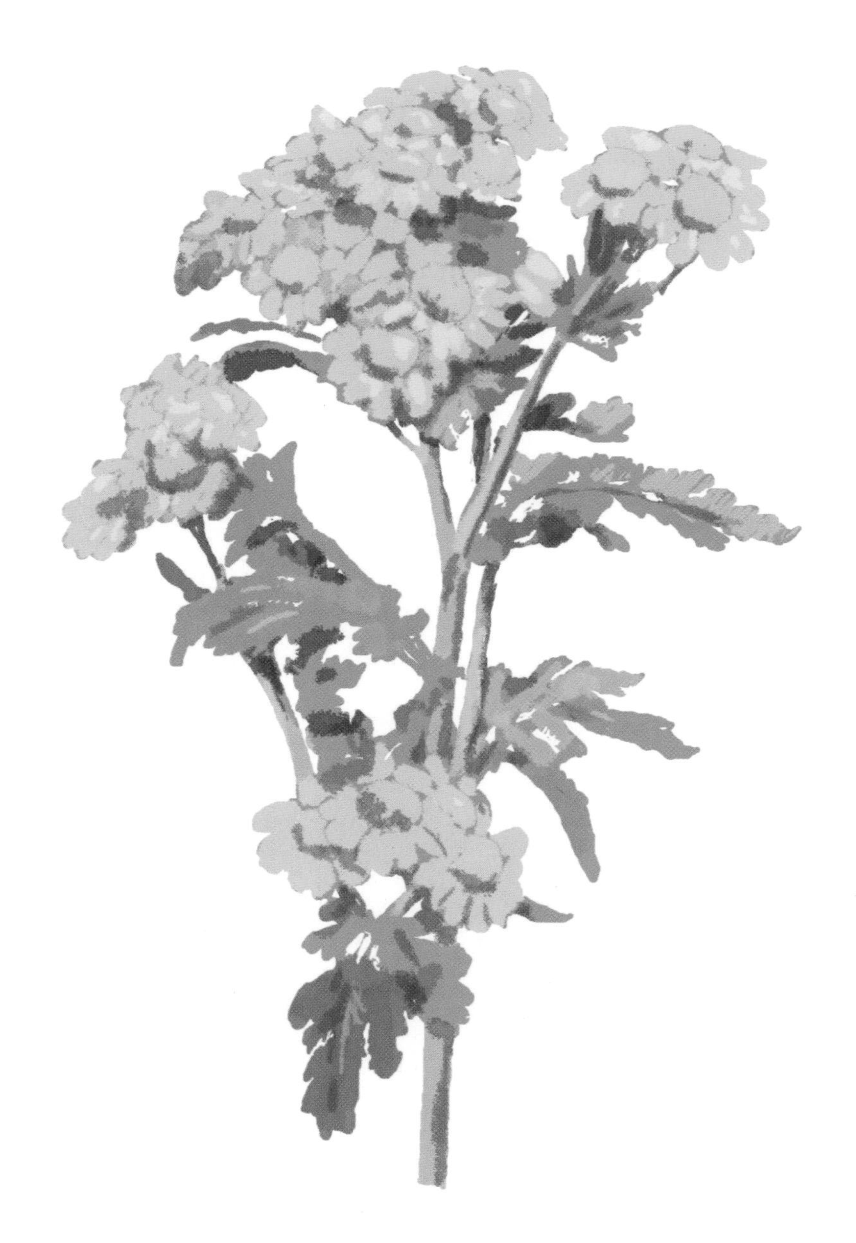

The pretty flowers are a bonus; the leaves and stalks contain feverfew's healing properties.

Feverfew
Tanacetum parthenium

There has been much research performed on this powerful herb, which has been shown to cure migraines and to treat minor fevers, rheumatism and arthritis.

Origins & Characteristics
Feverfew contains many chemicals, one of which (parthenolide) has the ability to block the action of serotonin, an inflammatory chemical released from special blood cells called platelets. Prostaglandins, hormone-like substances released from white blood cells, can aggravate migraines by affecting the blood circulation to the brain. These actions are blocked by feverfew extracts.

Parts Used
Leaves and stalks

Dosage
As a liquid tincture, take 20 drops twice daily.

Potential Benefits
- Acts as a migraine treatment
- Helps control minor fevers
- May be helpful in cases of joint pain and arthritis

Caution
Avoid during pregnancy. It is not advised to eat the fresh leaves because these may cause mouth ulcers in sensitive individuals.

Tansy
Tanacetum vulgare

Ever since medieval times, tansy has been used as an effective insect repellent. The leaves can act as a fly repellent when hung in the home or the flowers can be included in pot pourri. The name comes from the Greek word for immortality – *athanasia* – and tansy was used for embalming as it was thought to confer immortality to the deceased.

Origins & Characteristics

Tansy has a variety of effective therapeutic uses. It is a powerful emmenagogue, stimulating menstruation, as well as having good antiparasitic properties. This makes it useful for treating and eliminating roundworms and threadworms from the digestive tract. This herb also improves digestion and helps relieve dyspepsia. Applied externally, tansy can be used to treat scabies as well as help with rheumatism.

Parts Used

Leaves

Dosage

For external application, use as a compress to treat scabies and rheumatic joints.

Potential Benefits

- Stimulates menstruation
- Eliminates worms
- Improves digestion
- Relieves dyspepsia
- Helps treat rheumatism
- Helps treat scabies

Culinary Uses

Fresh leaves may be used in salads and egg dishes, but only use in small quantities.

Caution

Avoid using over a long period of time. Avoid during pregnancy. An overdose of tansy tea or oil can be fatal.

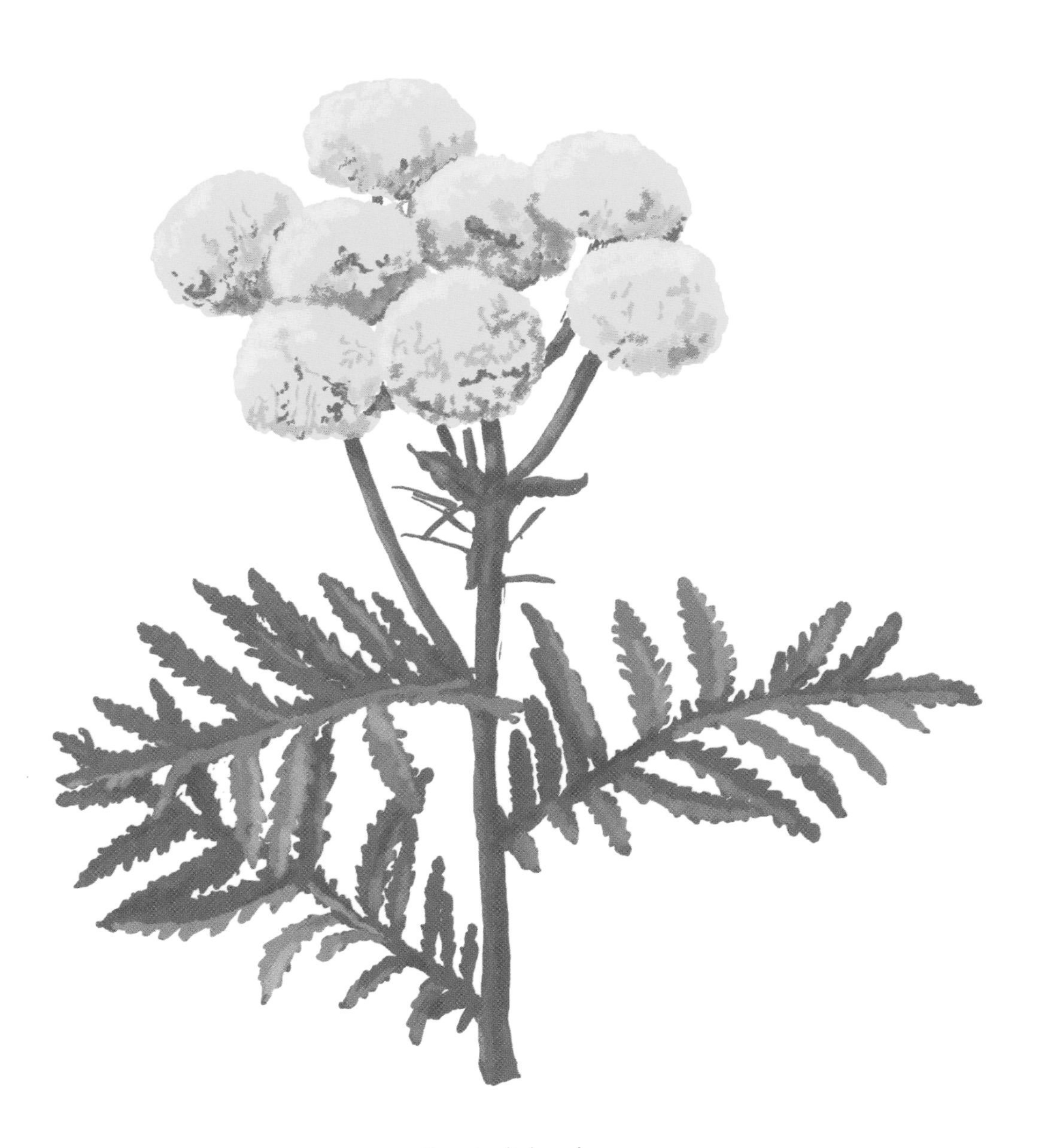

Tansy is a little used medicinal herb, but has many healing properties.

Dandelion
Taraxacum officinale

The dandelion first appeared in European medicine in 1480, having been used by the Chinese since A.D. 659. Dandelion acts as a diuretic, increasing the urine flow so much that early users often called it 'wet-the-bed'. Its high potassium content is thought to be responsible for this action.

Origins & Characteristics
High blood pressure has also been reduced by dandelion treatment thanks to its diuretic activity and potassium content. The liver and gallbladder can benefit from dandelion, which appears to enhance the function of these organs. For this reason it has been used for the treatment of hepatitis, gallstones, gout and skin problems, including eczema.

Parts Used
Whole plant

Dosage
As a liquid tincture, take 20 drops twice daily.

Potential Benefits
- Acts as a liver-stimulating agent
- Increases flow of bile
- Helps in skin conditions such as eczema
- Lowers blood pressure
- Increases urine flow (diuretic)
- Is a good source of potassium

Cosmetic Uses
Add an infusion of dandelion leaves to the bath to cleanse the skin.

Culinary Uses
Cook fresh leaves like spinach or add to a salad.

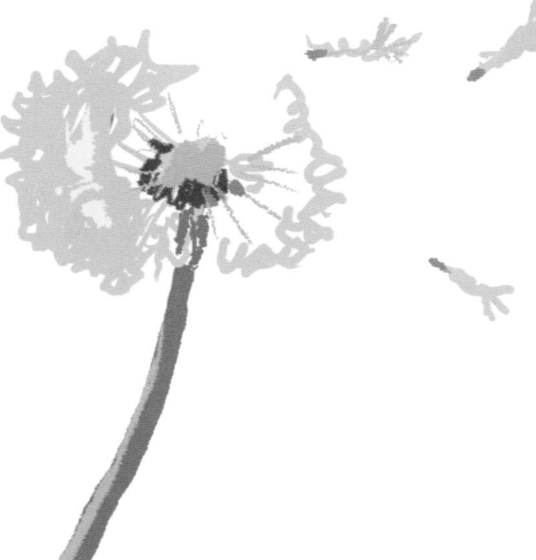

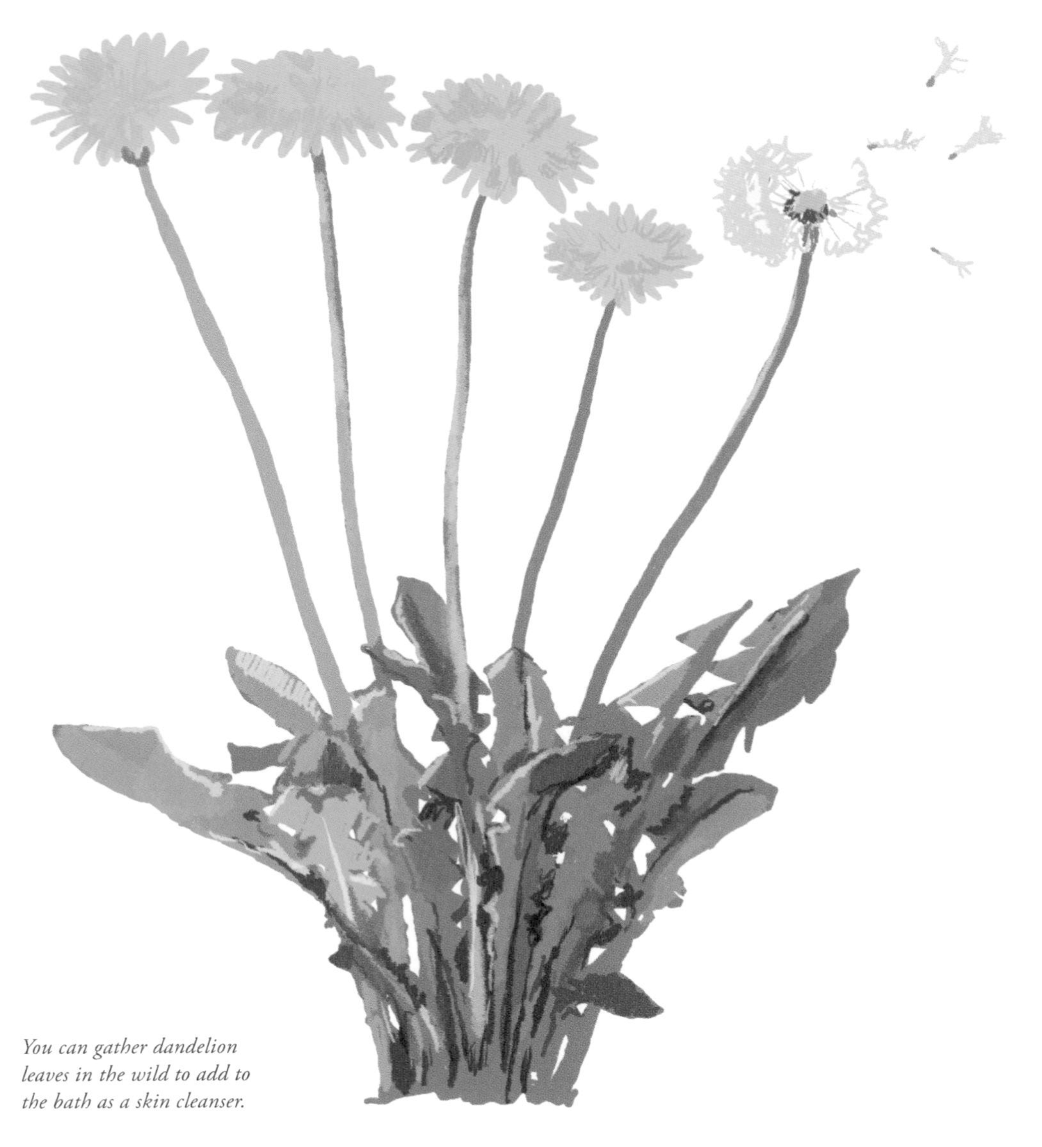

You can gather dandelion leaves in the wild to add to the bath as a skin cleanser.

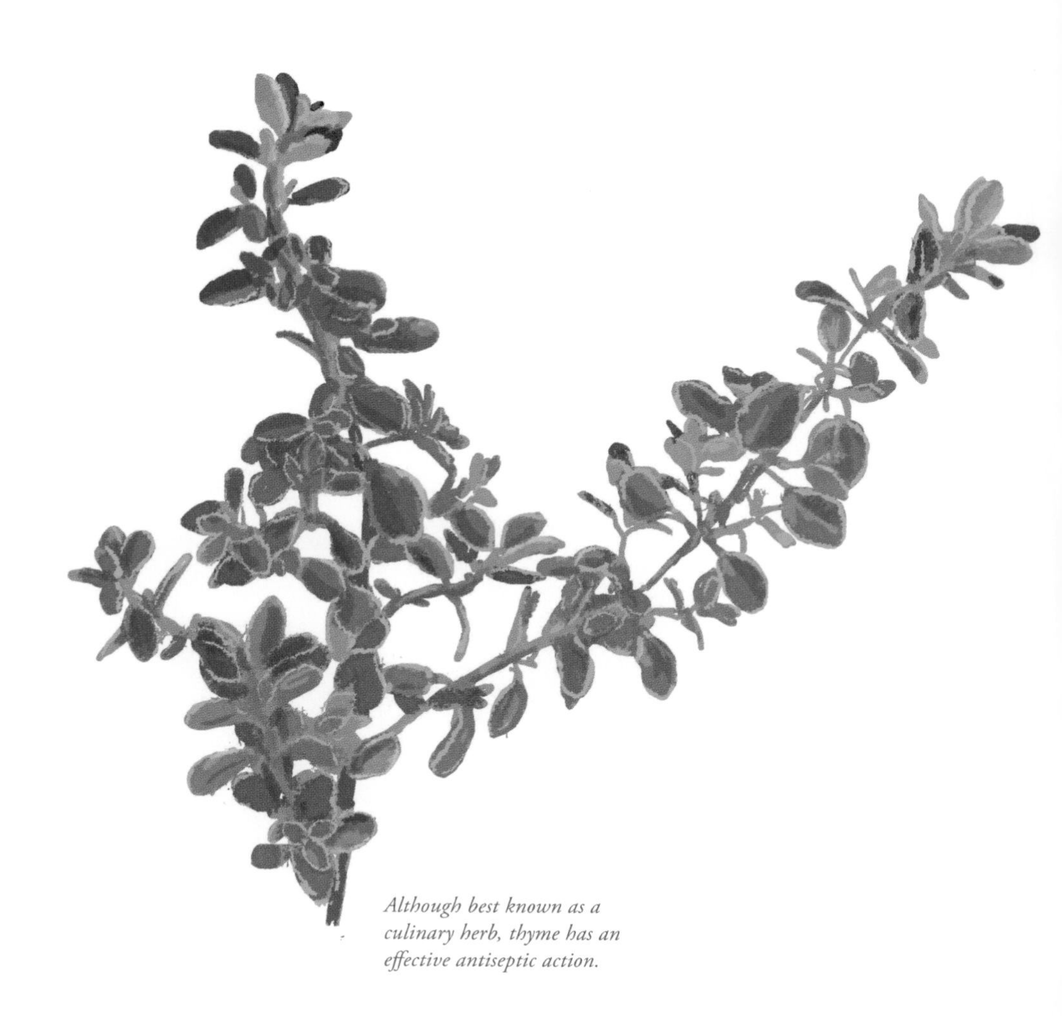

Although best known as a culinary herb, thyme has an effective antiseptic action.

Thyme
Thymus vulgaris

Thyme is another herb with valuable antiseptic properties, the active agent being thymol. Thyme is an herb with a long tradition of use in respiratory problems. It is taken internally for coughs and colds or more serious problems such as bronchitis and asthma.

Caution

Do not use the essential oil of thyme internally. Avoid using this herb during pregnancy.

Origins & Characteristics

The mucus-clearing ability of thyme makes it the appropriate remedy for chronic congestion when inflammation is a problem. Externally, thyme can soothe painful joints.

The aroma of thyme varies among species and depends on the concentrations of oils present in the plant.

Parts Used

Whole plant

Dosage

As a liquid tincture, take 20 drops twice daily.

For external application, use 6 drops of essential oil, mixed with 2 teaspoons of almond oil and apply to the desired area.

Potential Benefits

- Clears lung congestion and infections
- Helps reduce asthma symptoms
- Has an antiseptic action
- Relieves colds
- Soothes painful joints

Culinary Uses

Thyme is the basis of a *bouquet garni*, a bag or bundle of herbs used to flavour a dish while cooking. Try adding a little to soups, meat and fish dishes. Added to marinades, thyme provides a special flavour.

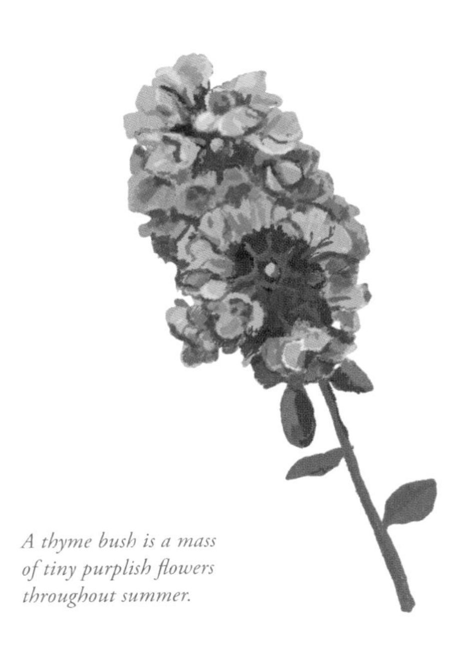

A thyme bush is a mass of tiny purplish flowers throughout summer.

Fenugreek
Trigonella foenum-graecum

As far back as 1500 B.C., fenugreek was being used and its effects documented in the writings of the ancient Egyptians. Its ability to reduce muscular spasm made it the herb of choice in menstrual cramps and labour pains. It was even used in ancient civilisations to induce childbirth.

Origins & Characteristics

Modern medicine has been interested in extracts of fenugreek since the isolation of two chemicals: trigonelline, a potential cancer treatment, and certain saponins that can be used in contraceptive preparations. The traditional use of this herb has been in the treatment of non-insulin-dependent diabetes, inflammation of the stomach, digestive problems and menstrual cramps. Fenugreek is also used to stimulate the flow of breast milk in nursing mothers. An external application can help arthritis.

Parts Used

Leaves and seeds

Dosage

As a liquid tincture, take 20 drops twice daily.

For external application, use as a poultice; mix freshly crushed seeds with a little water and apply as needed.

Potential Benefits

- Reduces menstrual cramps
- Can stimulate the flow of breast milk
- Improves digestion
- Assists in the balance of blood sugars
- Soothes arthritic joints

Culinary Uses

Use fenugreek seeds to add a spicy flavour to pea soups and to cooked carrots.

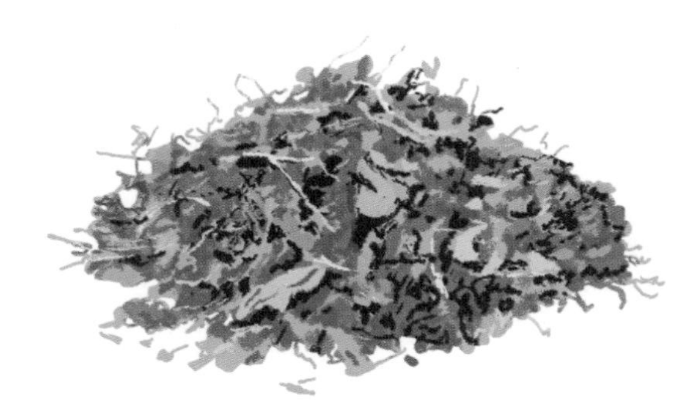

Fenugreek leaves are often used in Indian cooking.

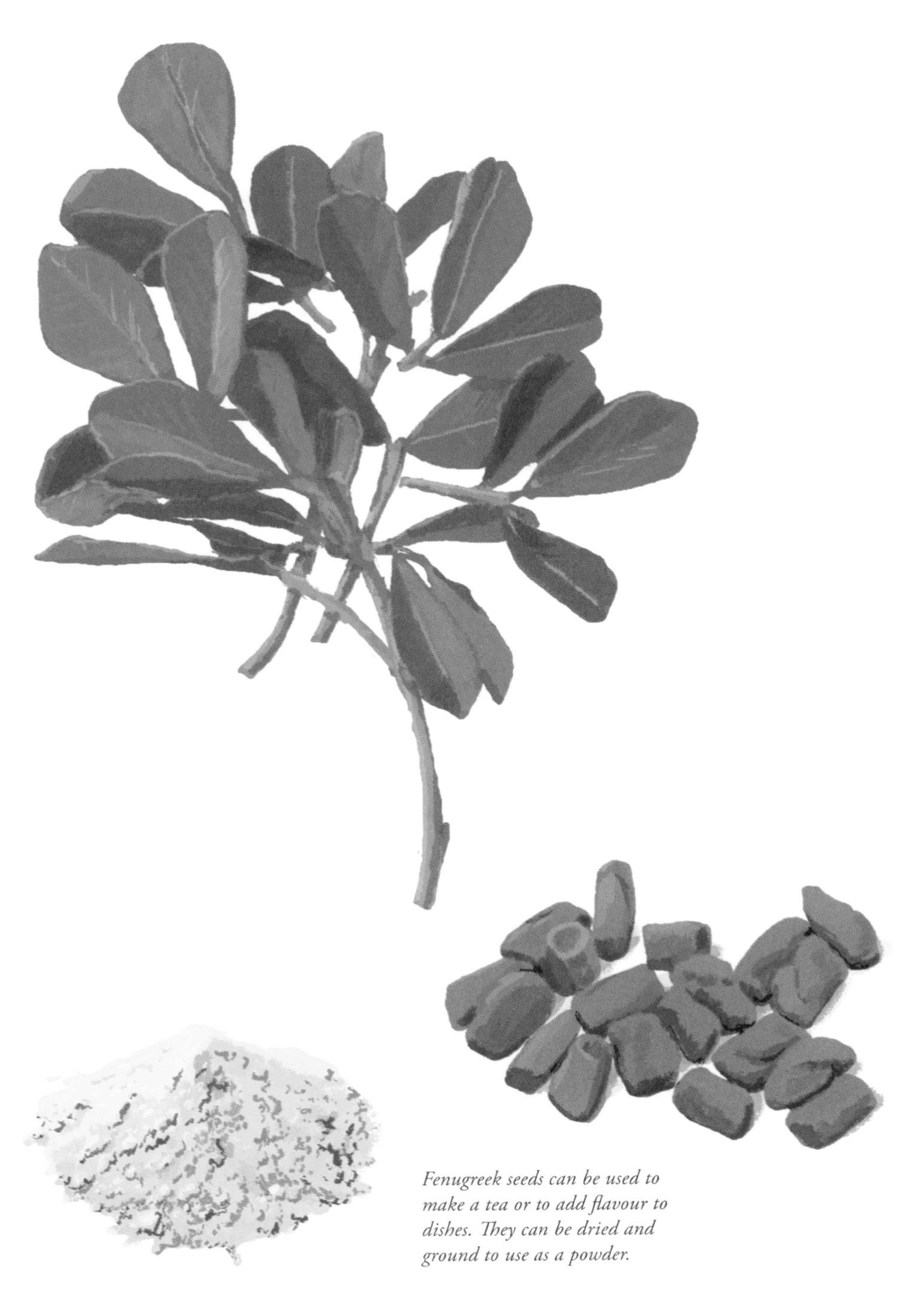

Fenugreek seeds can be used to make a tea or to add flavour to dishes. They can be dried and ground to use as a powder.

Coltsfoot
Tussilago farfara

Coltsfoot was used as far back as A.D. 23–79, when the leaves and roots were burned over coals and the smoke generated was taken as a remedy for persistent cough. During the classical period, coltsfoot was smoked for the treatment of asthma and lung congestion.

Origins & Characteristics

Coltsfoot has a licorice flavour. It is used for the control of spasms involving the respiratory system. As a cough expectorant, coltsfoot is quite effective, but its main application is to reduce inflammation associated with irritated mucous membranes in the respiratory tract. Externally, coltsfoot has a soothing effect on inflamed skin, especially eczema and dermatitis.

Parts Used

Flowers and leaves

Dosage

As a liquid tincture, take 20 drops twice daily after eating.

For external application, use coltsfoot leaves as a compress for eczema and dermatitis.

Potential Benefits

- Acts as a cough remedy and expectorant
- Helps control asthma
- Eases symptoms of bronchitis and laryngitis
- Has a soothing effect on inflamed skin

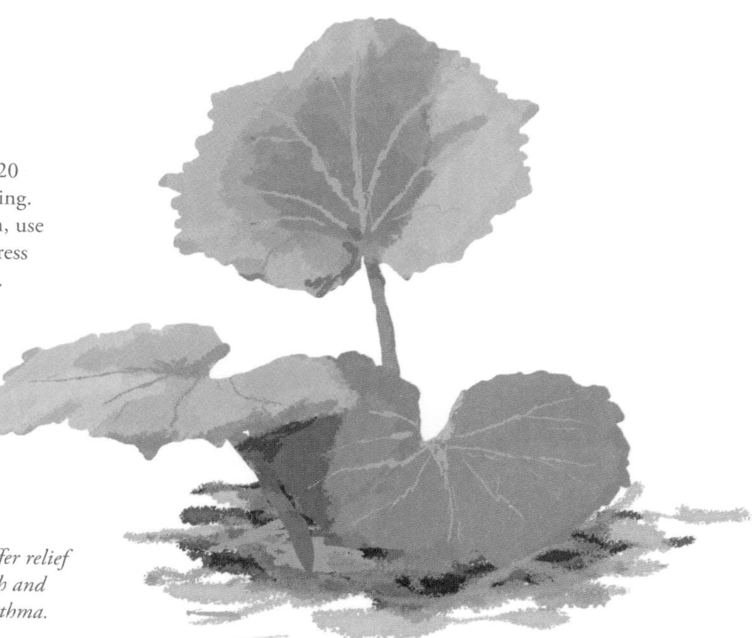

Coltsfoot leaves can offer relief from a persistent cough and even help to control asthma.

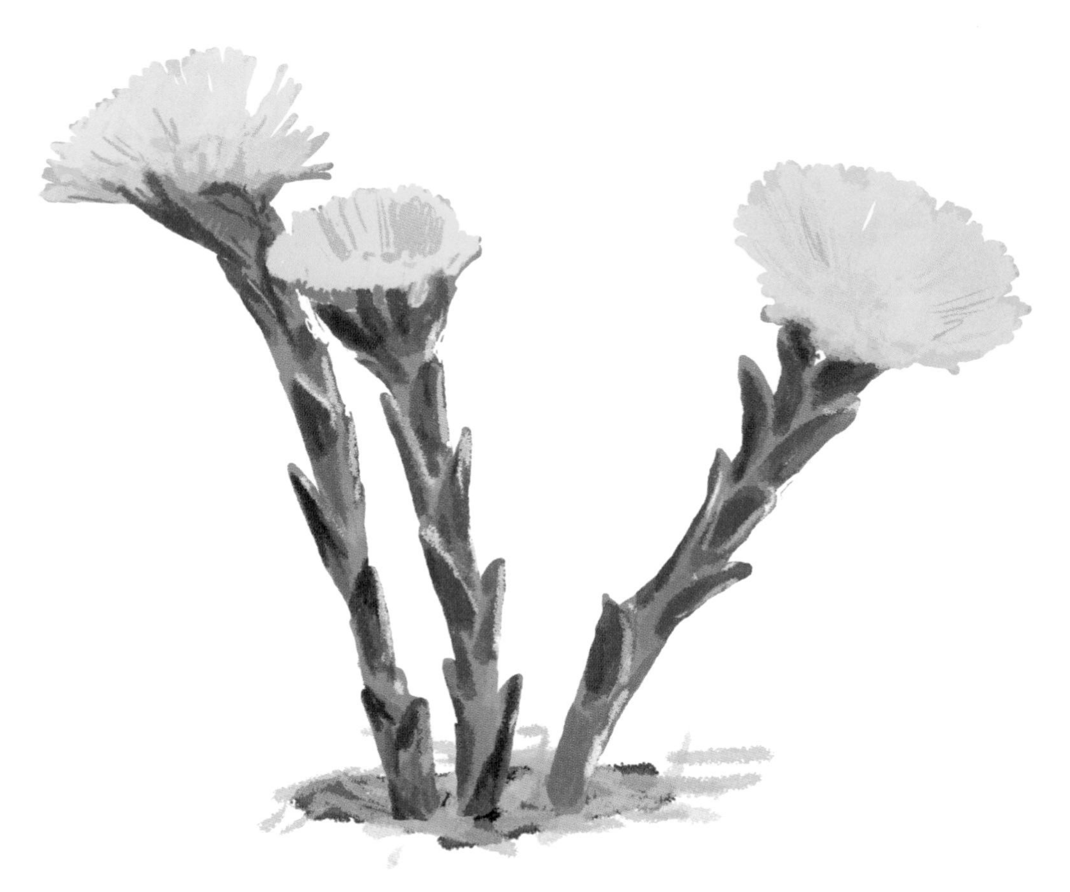

What initially look like scales on the flower stems of coltsfoot unfurl into leaves (left).

Sassafras Leaves
Umbellularia californica

A native plant of California, sassafras leaves were found to be a very effective insect repellent. The sassafras plant has a strong camphoraceous aroma, and it has been used as an inhalant for the treatment of headaches and sinus congestion.

Origins & Characteristics
Sassafras leaves have been used traditionally for the treatment of headache and neuralgia. They are bound to the painful area in the form of a poultice.

Parts Used
Leaves

Dosage
As an infusion, take 500–750ml (2 or 3 cups) daily.
As a liquid tincture, take 25 drops twice daily.

Potential Benefits
- Acts as a headache remedy
- Helps in cases of neuralgia

Culinary Uses
Try using in place of bay leaves in meat dishes or stews.

Caution
Do not use sassafras roots as they are carcinogenic.

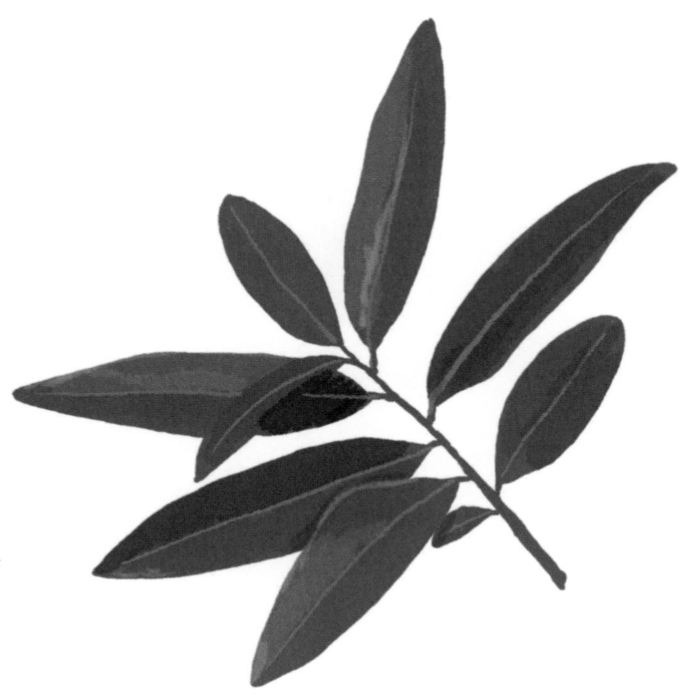

To treat a headache, try tying sassafras leaves to your painful head as a poultice.

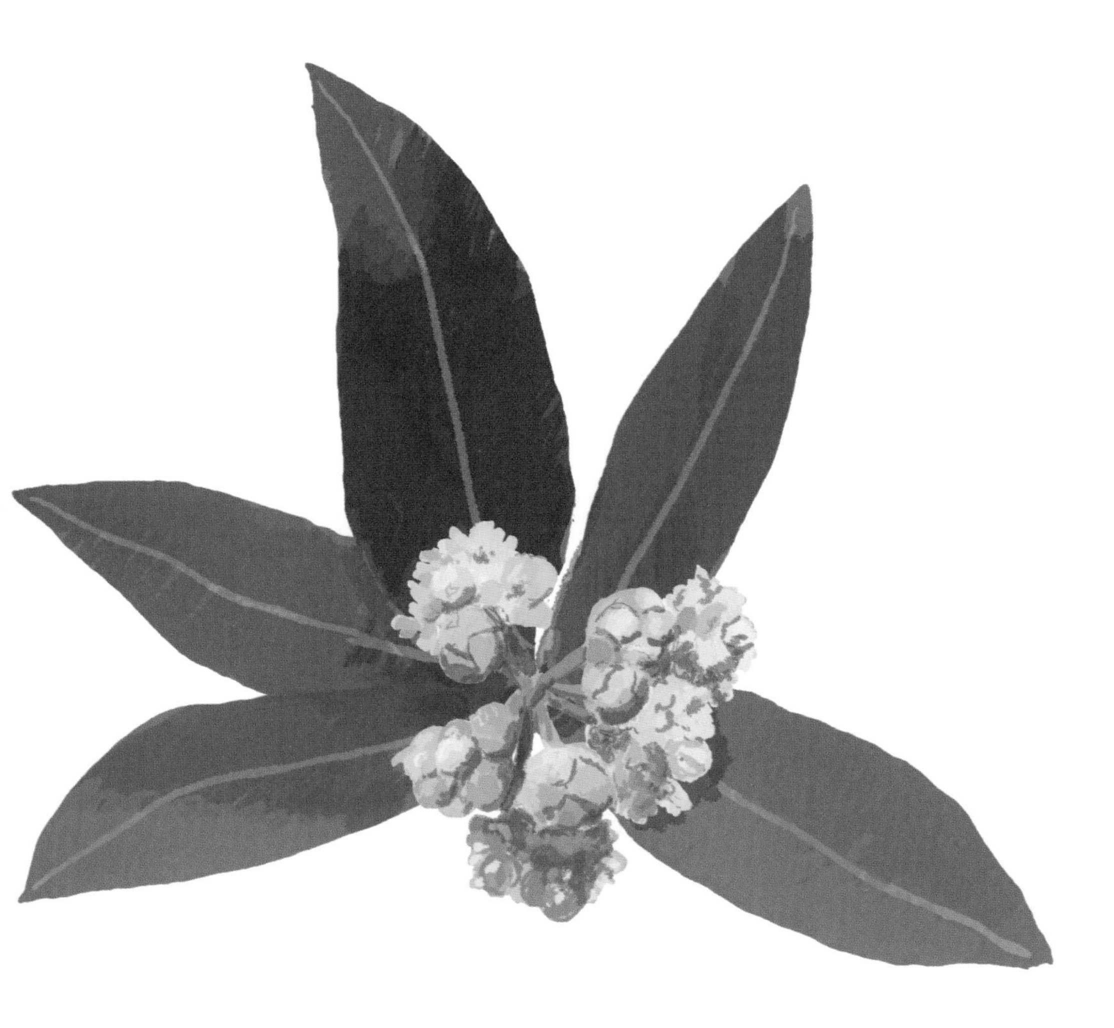

Sassafras leaves come from a large, hardwood tree which bears small, yellowish flowers.

Nettle
Urtica dioica

Nettle has been used since Roman times for treating rheumatic disease. The Romans would flail the inflamed joints with nettles to induce an inflammatory reaction that would calm down the disease. Nettles contain a rich source of nutrients, especially vitamins A, B and C, and minerals including silica.

Origins & Characteristics
The astringent properties of the herb can help reduce the blood flow, control bleeding and reduce blood pressure. It may be used to treat nosebleeds.

Taken internally, nettles can help rebalance the nutritional status of anemia sufferers. It may be helpful in controlling excessive menstrual bleeding.

Arthritis, gout and rheumatism can all be reduced by using nettles, probably due to their diuretic action.

Parts Used
Whole plant and leaves

Dosage
As a liquid tincture, take 20 drops twice daily.

Potential Benefits
- Reduces symptoms of arthritis and rheumatism
- Supports requirements needed to prevent anaemia
- Controls bleeding

Cosmetic Uses
Use in shampoo to help reduce dandruff.

Culinary Uses
Cook the young leaves like spinach or purée for soups.

Nettles can be made into wine or beer. Older leaves can be gritty and should not be used for cooking.

Caution
Do not use the uncooked plant for culinary purposes as it is poisonous and can cause kidney damage.

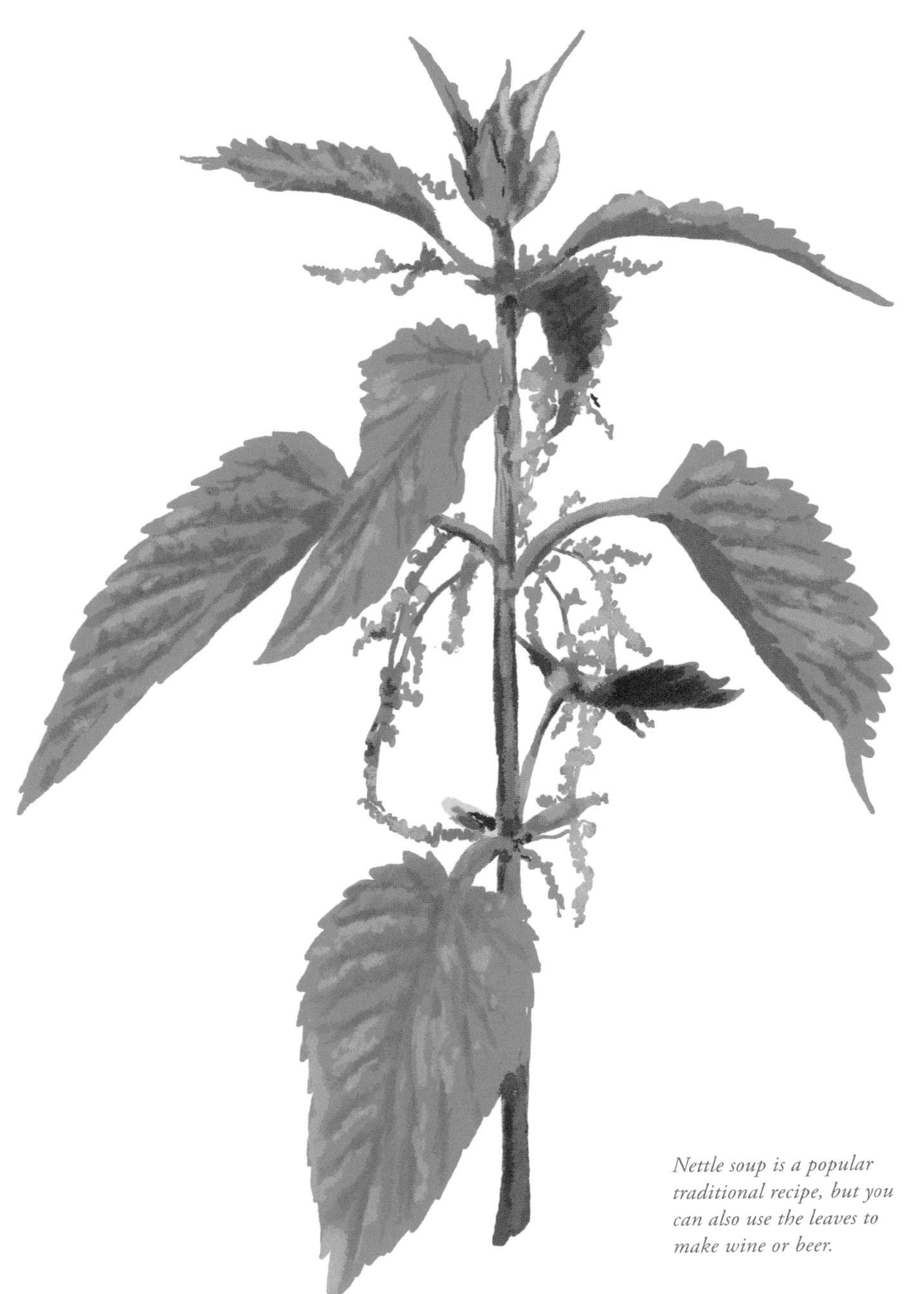

Nettle soup is a popular traditional recipe, but you can also use the leaves to make wine or beer.

Cranberry
Vaccinium macrocarpon

Cranberries contain about 80 per cent water and have a high vitamin C content. Their citric acid levels are very high – higher even than that of lemons. The healing properties of cranberries date back to the seventeenth century, when they were used for the treatment of stomach and liver problems. Cranberries have become the herb of choice for the treatment of bladder infections.

Origins & Characteristics

Studies have located a natural polymer, arbutin, that actually prevents the bacteria from sticking to the wall of the bladder and urinary tract. An earlier theory suggested that cranberries made the urine acidic, which killed bacteria, but this theory has been replaced by the finding that bacteria actually lose their foothold on the walls of the urinary system in the presence of cranberry extracts.

Parts Used

Fruits

Dosage

Take 2 tablets (100mg) of dried berries twice daily in acute phase, reducing to 1 tablet (50mg) over the following month.

Drink 1 teaspoon of cranberry powder (commercially prepared) in 150ml (5fl oz) of water twice daily until symptoms ease, reducing to ½ teaspoon for the next month.

Potential Benefits

- Acts as a cystitis treatment
- Acts as a urinary cleanser

Culinary Uses

The fruits can be added to preserves, desserts and salads. They make a traditional jelly-like condiment to accompany roast turkey at Christmas.

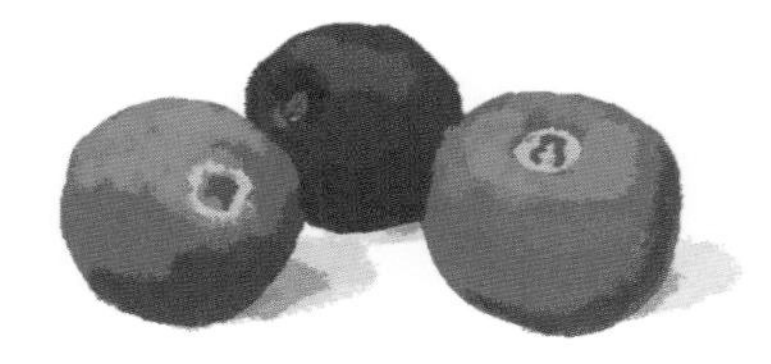

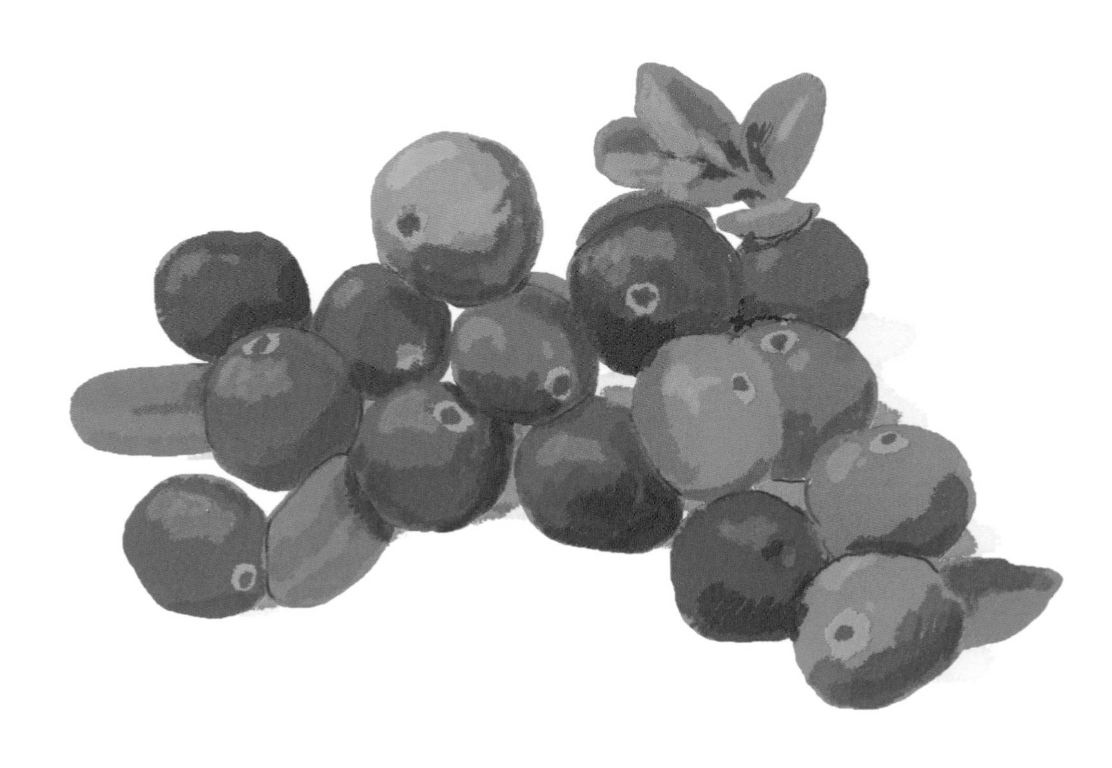

Cranberries have two well-known uses: as a sauce to go with turkey and a treatment for cystitis.

Bilberry
Vaccinium myrtillus

Bilberry is full of beneficial phytochemicals. Blood sugar levels are improved by the substances known as glucoquinones, while other agents called anthrocyanosides keep blood circulation flowing by dilating blood vessels. The species of bilberry *Vaccinium myrtillus* contains a unique substance (arbutin) that has powerful antiseptic effects on the urinary system and has been used as an effective natural cystitis treatment.

Origins & Characteristics
During World War II, British RAF pilots received preserves made from bilberry to improve their night vision. Recent studies have confirmed that bilberry extract can regenerate visual purple (the chemical that keeps night vision healthy) and, therefore, improve vision.

Parts Used
Leaves and fruits

Dosage
As a liquid tincture, take 20 drops twice daily.

Potential Benefits
- Improves vision
- Stabilises blood sugar levels
- Acts as an effective cystitis remedy

Culinary Uses
The fruits may be added to salads and incorporated into desserts or used to make preserves.

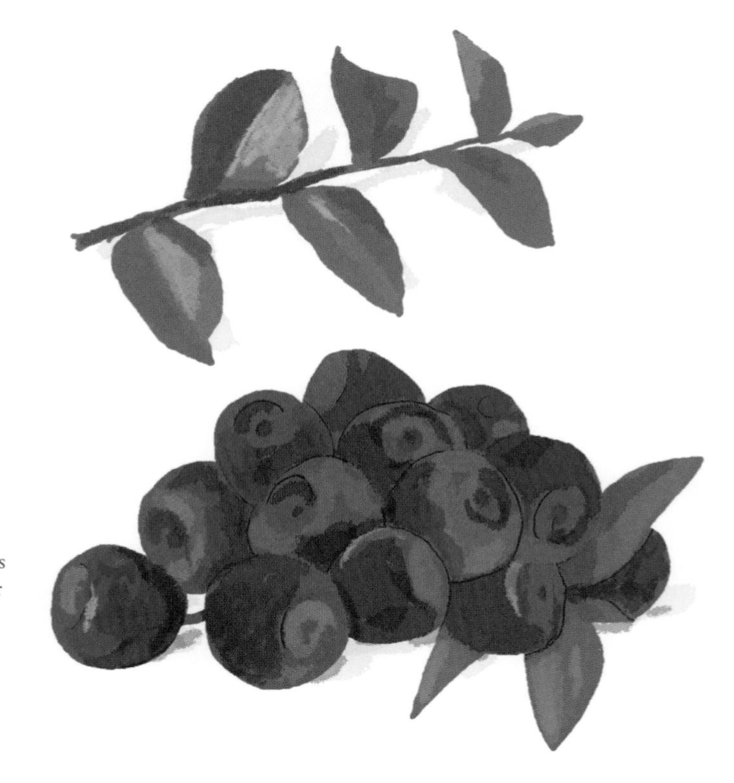

Bilberries can help to improve night vision.

Valerian
Valeriana officinalis

The name valerian is derived from the Latin word *valere* meaning 'to be well' and it helps by inducing a restful sleep and relaxation, allowing the body to divert its healing powers to where they are most needed.

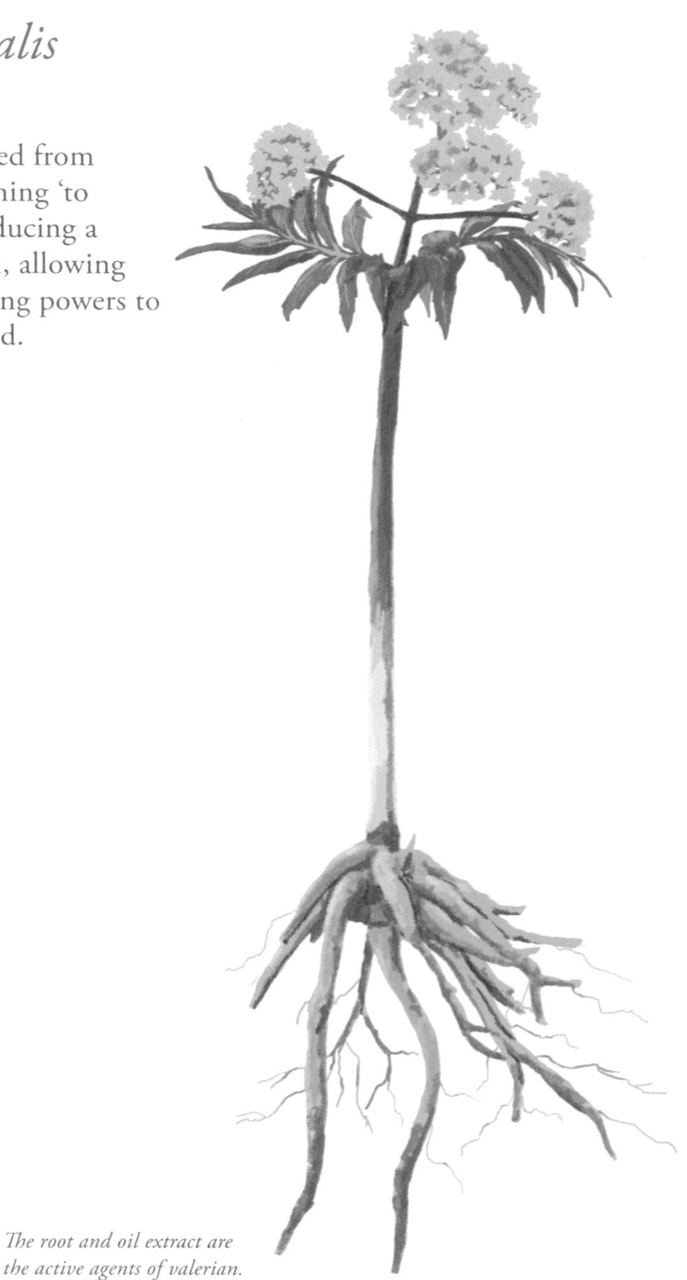

Origins & Characteristics
The traditional uses of this herb include treating hysteria, cramps, indigestion, high blood pressure, painful menstruation, palpitations and, of course, insomnia. Valerian may be combined with passionflower for a deeper sedative action, or it can be combined with licorice or hyssop and used as a cough expectorant. This herb can also help treat mouth ulcers when used as a mouthwash.

Parts Used
Rhizome, roots and oil extract

Dosage
As a sleep aid, take 25 drops of liquid tincture at bedtime. As a mouthwash, use a cooled infusion.

Potential Benefits
- Acts as a calming agent
- Induces a restful sleep
- Helps in panic attacks
- Reduces muscular tension
- Aids in menstrual cramps

The root and oil extract are the active agents of valerian.

Mullein
Verbascum thapus

Mullein has been used in folkloric medicine to treat respiratory disorders including coughs, congestion and asthma. It was traditionally used to treat serious wasting conditions, such as tuberculosis, and was associated with witchcraft. It was thought that witches used the hairs on top of the leaves to make potions.

Origins & Characteristics

The stems of mullein were also dipped in tallow and used as torches by the Greeks and Romans. Mullein has good expectorant and anti-inflammatory properties and can be used to soothe dry and irritating coughs as well as help expel phlegm.

Parts Used

Leaves

Dosage

As an infusion, add 2 teaspoons of dried leaves to 250ml (9fl oz) boiling water and let stand for 5 minutes.

Take a liquid tincture made from the flowers for coughs and sore throats.

Take a leaf tincture for eliminating phlegm.

Potential Benefits

- Soothes dry and irritated coughs
- Acts as a mild sedative
- Has a mild diuretic action
- Has an expectorant action
- Has an anti-inflammatory action

Cosmetic Uses

Use the dried flowers infused in water to make a hair rinse to lighten hair.

Mullein flowers rise in a spike from a clump of leaves.

Vervain
Verbena officinalis

Vervain has a long history of medicinal uses, especially treating nervous disorders. Taken internally, vervain can help depression that is often present after an illness and can help to treat stress-related headaches and migraines. This herb contains bitters that stimulate the liver and help relieve hepatitis and jaundice. It also stimulates the digestive system and improves digestion.

Origins & Characteristics
Vervain has a diuretic action, which makes it useful for relieving fluid retention. This herb is an effective emmenagogue. Taken as a tea at bedtime, it acts as a mild sedative. Vervain can be used to soothe inflamed eyes. This herb can also be used to treat insect bites and sprains.

Parts Used
Leaves

Dosage
As a tea, add 2 teaspoons of dried leaves to 250ml (9fl oz) of boiling water and let stand for 5 minutes before drinking.

For external application, use as a diluted infusion for soothing inflamed eyes. Vervain can also be used externally as a poultice for insect bites and minor injuries and as an ointment for treating eczema.

Potential Benefits
- Helps depression
- Improves digestion
- Alleviates nervous disorders
- Helps relieve hepatitis and jaundice
- Stimulates menstruation
- Has a diuretic action
- Has a mild sedative action
- Helps soothe inflamed eyes

Caution
Avoid during pregnancy as vervain acts as a stimulant to the uterus.

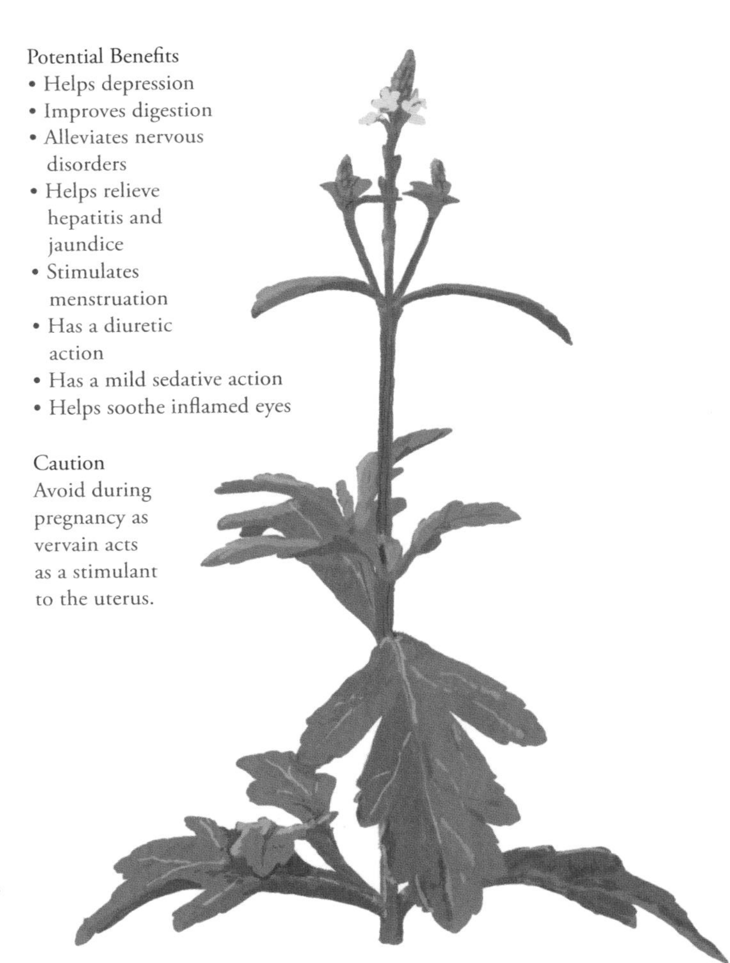

Vervain is a tall and slender plant. Its leaves are harvested and used for medicinal purposes.

Crampbark
Viburnum opulus

Crampbark and its close relative stagbush (*Viburnum prunifolium*) have been used since colonial times as treatments for painful menstruation. Contained within the plant are botanical substances that relax the uterus and, therefore, reduce the pains associated with menstrual cramps. The plant has also been used in cases of threatened miscarriage and high blood pressure.

Parts Used
Bark

Dosage
As a liquid tincture, take 20 drops twice daily.

Potential Benefits
- Reduces pains associated with menstruation and uterine cramps
- May help prevent miscarriage
- Helps lower high blood pressure

Caution
Do not eat the uncooked fruits, as they are poisonous.

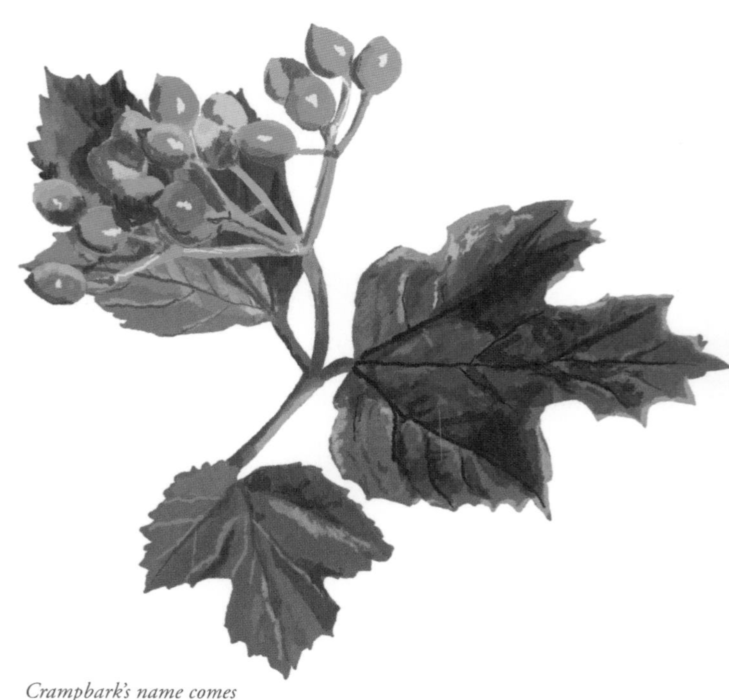

Crampbark's name comes from its soothing benefit for menstruation pain.

Yucca
Yucca gloriosa

The chemical saponin contained within the yucca has been shown to affect toxins absorbed by the stomach bacteria. It is these toxins that may be responsible for the destruction of joint cartilage, so yucca, in blocking the uptake, may hold possible therapeutic applications in the treatment of arthritis.

Origins & Characteristics
The observation that yucca can help to treat arthritis has been supported by the traditional use of yucca by Native Americans for the treatment of inflamed joints and rheumatism.

Parts Used
Sap

Dosage
Take 2 tablets (100mg) of dried sap daily.

Potential Benefits
- Reduces inflammation
- Eases symptoms of rheumatism
- May be a possible arthritis remedy

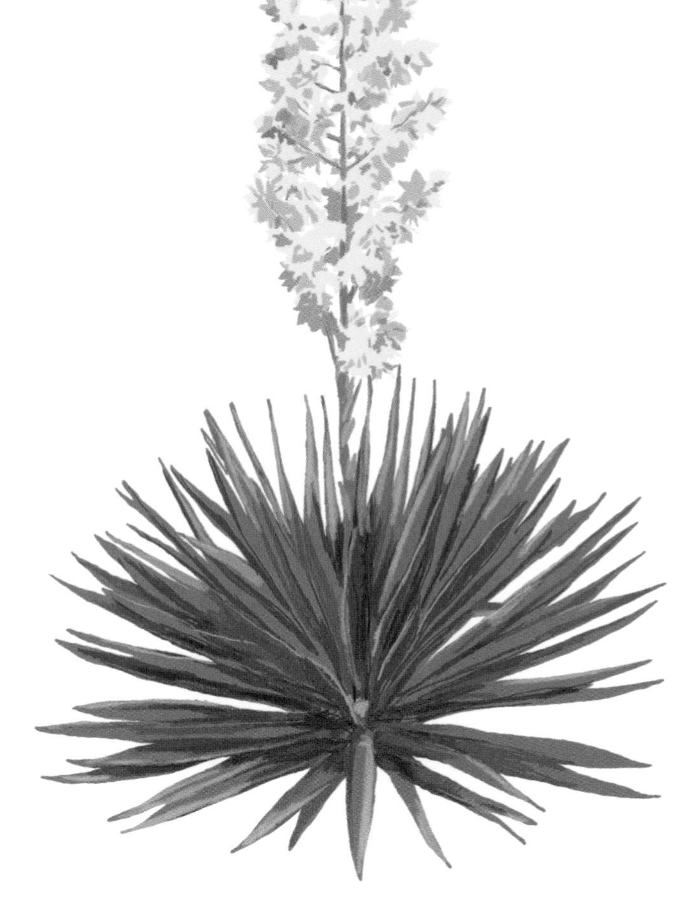

The yucca is a stately plant, particularly when in flower. Its sap is used to treat joint pain.

Ginger
Zingiber officinale

Ginger's active agent is gingerol. On drying, gingerols break down into chemicals called shogaols, which are twice as potent, meaning that dried ginger is more pungent than fresh. Ginger's main effect on humans is to reduce nausea and motion sickness. It has become a popular herb for the treatment of morning sickness associated with pregnancy. Its safety in recommended doses is good, but excessive intake can be dangerous. This herb also promotes gastric secretions and is useful in treating flatulence.

Origins & Characteristics
Ginger has been used as a traditional treatment for skin irritations, both applied externally and by internal dosage. For colds and flu, ginger extract has a warming effect and can boost the immune response to infection. Ginger has a powerful diaphoretic action and induces sweating. It can also be used as a gargle to relieve sore throats.

Parts Used
Rhizome and oil extract

Dosage
As a liquid tincture, take 25 drops twice daily.

As a tea, crush a slice of fresh ginger root and add to the infusion.

Potential Benefits
- Acts as an antinausea remedy
- Helps in morning sickness
- Reduces cold and flu symptoms
- Reduces sweating
- Helps relieve flatulence
- Boosts the immune response

Culinary Uses
Add a couple of slices of freshly chopped ginger root to a stir-fry, curry or gingerbread mixture for an extra-fresh flavour, or add to salad dressings.

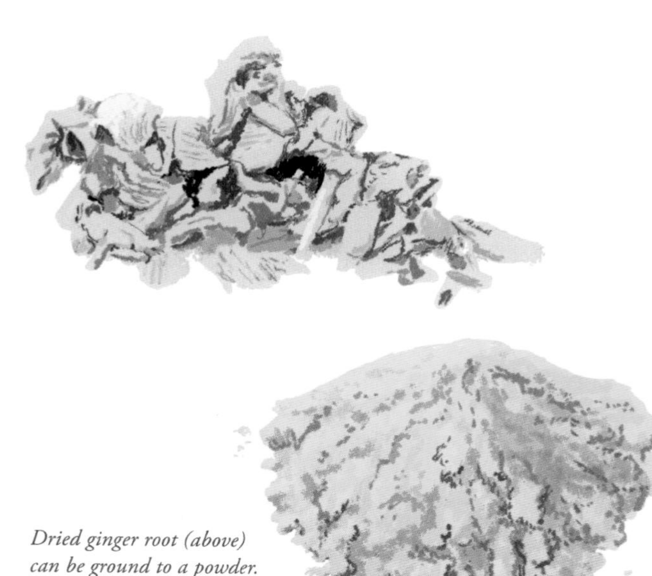

Dried ginger root (above) can be ground to a powder.

Ginger Dressing for a Spicy Fruit Salad

- 50g (2oz) sugar
- 150ml (5fl oz) water
- 150ml (5fl oz) ginger wine
- 2 pieces of chopped stem ginger
- finely grated rind and juice of 1½ limes

Put the sugar and water in a saucepan and heat gently, stirring, until the sugar has dissolved. Bring to a boil, then simmer for 1 minute without stirring. Remove from the heat and add the remaining ingredients. Pour over prepared fruit and leave to cool. Chill before serving.

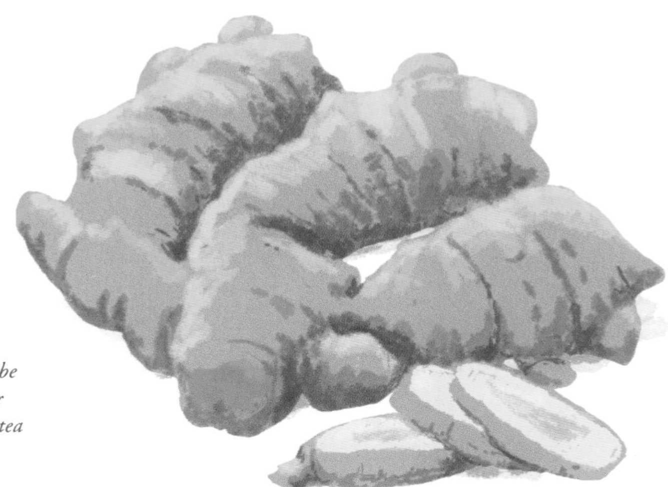

Fresh ginger root should be peeled before use. Slice or grate the root to make a tea or for use in cooking.

Herbal Remedies

The healing properties of some plants have been recognised for thousands of years – Hippocrates compiled a book of more than 400 medicinal herbs in around 400 B.C. and many of them remain in common usage today, in conjunction with conventional medicine. Each of the entries in the Directory of Herbs includes a list of the ailments that particular herb can help to treat or relieve; these pages offer more detailed advice for combatting common problems in children, adults and the elderly, and for relief from conditions such as stress, menopause and pregnancy.

CAUTION

Always consult a health-care professional before embarking on a programme of self-treatment. Herbal medicines are effective and safe when used correctly and every effort has been made to make this book as accurate and as informative as possible, but the advice contained within is no replacement for professional guidance.

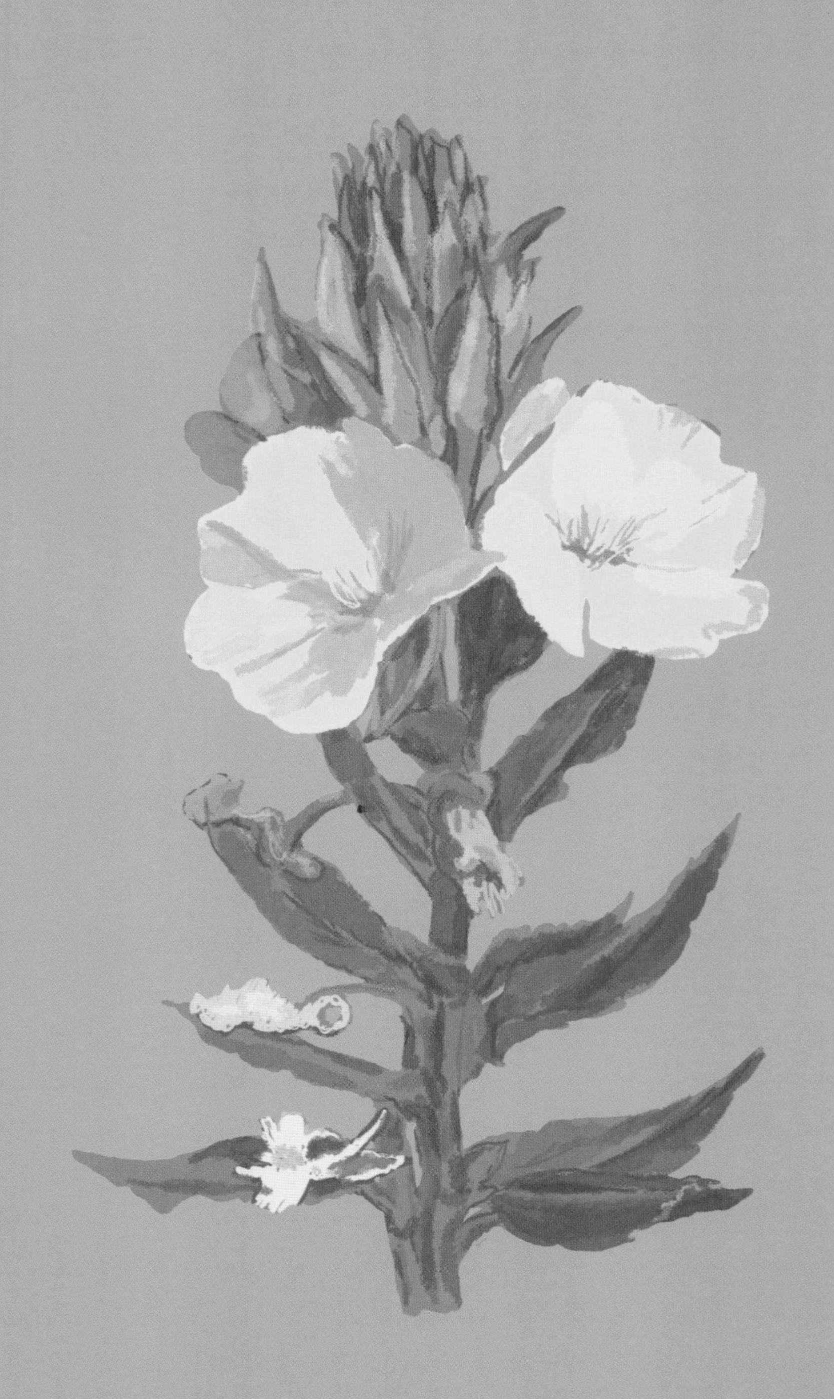

Children

There are many gentle herbal remedies that can offer soothing relief to children suffering from a range of common ailments, though they are best used alongside conventional medical treatments and with the advice of your pharmacist or family doctor.

FEVER

A fever is not always a bad thing, but keeping a close watch on the child's temperature is vital. The average body temperature is 37.0°C (98.6°F). A lower temperature is suggestive of shock or excessive cooling if you are sponging your child down with cold water, or it could be a sign that the temperature is going to increase soon, possibly up to 39.8°C (103°F) or more. Temperatures up to 38.8°C (101°F) are thought of as moderate fever; when this rises to 39.2–40.3°C (102–104°F) or more, it is considered to be seriously high, and seeking prompt medical attention is strongly advised.

If your child has a fever but is not sweating, try a natural sweat-inducing agent (known as a diaphoretic). A hot tea made from elder or chamomile can break a fever very effectively.

During the entire illness, doses of echinacea should be given at regular intervals to assist in the stimulation of the immune system. Its antiviral and antibacterial properties are other factors that make this the best extract for all illnesses.

UPSET STOMACH AND DIARRHOEA

All children from time to time suffer from diarrhoea and stomach pains often accompanied by a mild fever. This may be caused by an infection, food poisoning, new food in the diet (often rich foods), overexcitement and fright, very cold or chilled foods, overeating, too much sun and mental or physical distress.

For diarrhoea, try a tincture of dandelion or tormentil. As the upset stomach slowly improves, the appetite may take a little while to return to normal; if this is the case, try a dose of centaury.

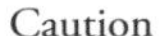

Caution

Diarrhoea can be life threatening. If the diarrhoea does not appear to improve and the child is becoming dehydrated, seek urgent medical attention.

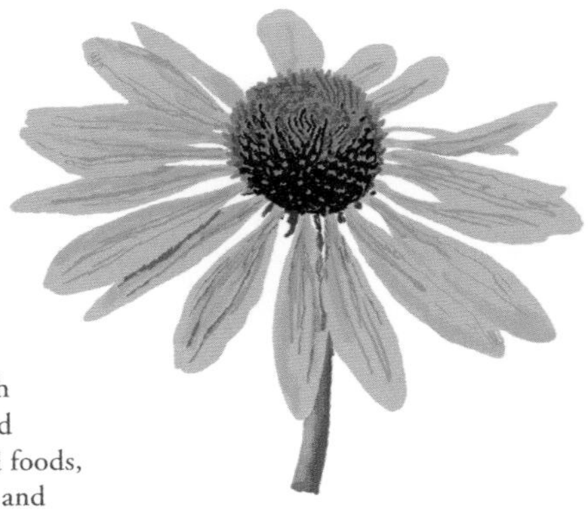

Extract of echinacea helps to boost the immune system.

Rehydration Formula

You will need:

- 250ml (9fl oz) water
- 1 tsp sugar
- pinch of baking soda
- pinch of salt

Boil the water, and, as it cools, add the sugar, a generous pinch of baking soda and a smaller pinch of salt. Stir until all of the ingredients have dissolved and give to the child when the formula is cold.

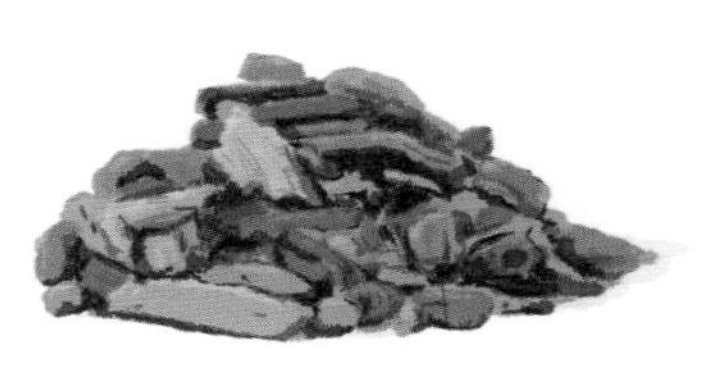

Liquid extract is produced from pieces of echinacea root.

COMMON CHILDHOOD AILMENTS

Chicken pox To ease the symptoms of skin irritation, try applying aloe vera salve or chamomile lotion. Taking a tea made from yarrow, chamomile, or goldenseal may also help.

Common Cold There is no cure for the common cold, but you can control many symptoms and, with luck, prevent your child from catching colds regularly. A daily dose of echinacea is essential, along with plenty of vitamin C-rich foods.

For a persistent cough, try sage tea, or for excessive mucus, a tea made from fenugreek or ginger can be very effective. A tincture of goldenseal is advisable during the infectious period to assist in fighting the infection.

Measles A tea made from yarrow, with the addition of a few drops of echinacea tincture, can be very beneficial. To stimulate the appetite when the worst of the disease is over, try a tincture of barberry.

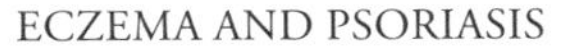

ECZEMA AND PSORIASIS

Both eczema and psoriasis are aggravated by stress and anxiety. The underlying reason for this is not known, but stress does increase the levels of certain hormones known to stimulate the circulation to the skin, which inflames an already irritated condition.

The irritation can be related to an imbalance in inflammatory chemicals, such as histamines, and dry flakiness. Skin inflammation is best approached by optimising fatty acid metabolism. There are many essential fatty acids, but the most important to the skin appear to be gamma linoleic acid (GLA) and the omega 3 and 6 oils.

Derived from borage seed and evening primrose seeds, GLA is probably the best known of all the essential fatty acids.

The omega 3 and 6 oils are found in fish and fish oils, linseeds, marine algae and meat from marine mammals such as seals and whales. Linseed oil contains both GLA and the omega 3 and 6 oils in one balanced form.

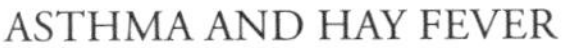

ASTHMA AND HAY FEVER

Herbal remedies such as Chinese skullcap, licorice, garlic and angelica commonly feature in the management of childhood asthma and hay fever.

Garlic has the ability to prevent a special enzyme (lipoxygenase) from working. The enzyme activates an important part of the inflammatory response, which is prevented by supplementation with garlic extract.

Angelica is especially effective in those individuals suffering from allergies to pollen, dust and animal dander. These allergens play an important role in generation of symptoms in hay fever and asthma.

Licorice also has anti-inflammatory and anti-allergy activity with a cortisone-like action. Steroids are widely used in the long-term management of asthma. Licorice extract has none of the side effects of steroids, but it does have many of the benefits. The inflammatory aspect of asthma can be managed using this extract.

Chinese skullcap has been used for its anti-inflammatory properties in the management of arthritis for many years. The herb contains high levels of flavonoids that work in a similar way to some anti-asthmatic drugs.

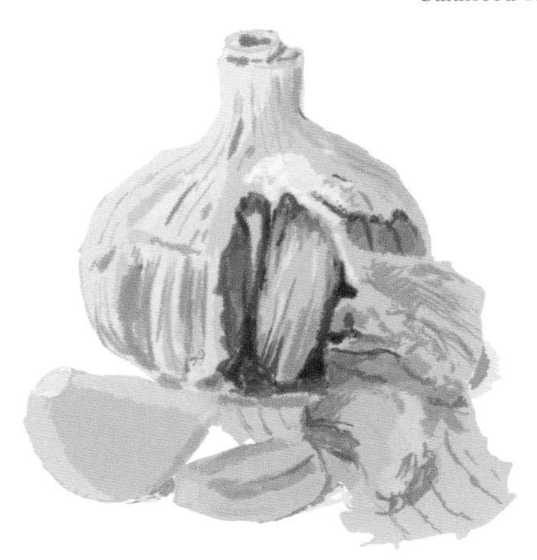

Garlic is widely used in herbal medicine. It can help to prevent lung infections – a great benefit to asthma sufferers.

COMMON PROBLEMS AND REMEDIES

Colic
- Extract of dill (*Anethum graveolens*)
- Fennel water (*Foeniculum vulgare*)
- Tincture of ginger (*Zingiber officinale*)
- Tincture of cloves (*Syzygium aromaticum*)

Constipation
- Extract of licorice (*Glycyrrhiza glabra*)
- Tincture of barberry (*Berberis vulgaris*)

Cough
- Elder syrup (*Sambucus nigra*)
- Tincture of plantain (*Plantago major*)
- Tea made from marshmallow (*Althaea officinalis*)

Cough with Phlegm
- Tincture of echinacea (*Echinacea purpura*)
- Tea made from ginger (*Zingiber officinale*) and fennel (*Foeniculum vulgare*) with honey

Cradle Cap
- Tincture of burdock (*Arctium lappa*)
- Tincture of nettle (*Urtica dioica*)
- Tincture of dandelion (*Taraxacum officinale*)
- Plantago ointment (*Plantago major*)
- Olive oil (*Olea europaea*)

Nappy Rash
- Zinc and castor oil cream
- Calendula ointment (*Calendula officinalis*)

Earache
- Tincture of hops (*Humulus lupulus*)
- Tincture of St. John's wort (*Hypericum perforatum*)
- Tincture of goldenseal (*Hydrastis canadensis*)
- Tincture of echinacea (*Echinacea purpura*)
- Tincture of plantain (*Plantago major*)

Nasal Congestion
- Tea made from hyssop (*Hyssopus officinalis*)
- Tincture of hyssop (*Hyssopus officinalis*)
- Tincture of goldenseal (*Hydrastis canadensis*)
- Extract of garlic (*Allium sativum*)

Sleeping Problems
- Tincture of lemon balm (*Melissa officinalis*)
- Tea made from lemon balm (*Melissa officinalis*)
- Tincture of valerian (*Valeriana officinalis*)
- Tincture of hops (*Humulus lupulus*)

Sore Throat
- Tincture of marshmallow (*Althaea officinalis*)
- Tincture of plantain (*Plantago major*)
- Tincture of elder (*Sambucus nigra*)
- Tincture of echinacea (*Echinacea purpura*)

Teething
- Tincture of chamomile (*Anthemis nobilis*)
- Marshmallow syrup (*Althea officinalis*)

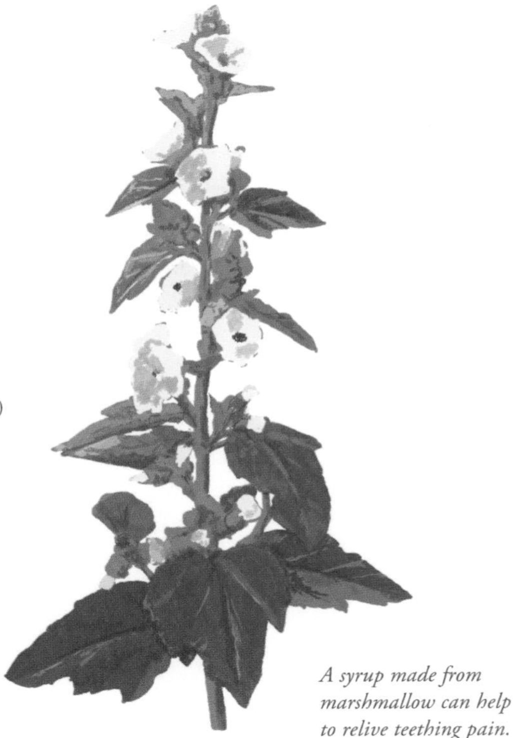

A syrup made from marshmallow can help to relive teething pain.

Young People and Adults

Childhood diseases are replaced by a new set of common ailments in adulthood. Patients suffering from persistent conditions, such as premenstrual syndrome, cystitis and irritable bowel syndrome, can often find relief in some simple herbal remedies.

PREMENSTRUAL SYNDROME (PMS)

It has been estimated that up to 75 per cent of women suffer from some form of premenstrual anxiety. Other symptoms, such as food cravings, weight gain and depression also occur to varying degrees. There are many safe, natural ways to conquer PMS.

Anxiety tends to be due to a hormone imbalance, namely excessive oestrogen and low progesterone levels. The high oestrogen has a blocking effect on vitamin B6, inhibiting the liver production of serotonin and altering the ability to balance blood sugar levels. A rise and fall of sugars is partly responsible for mood elevation and depression.

Herbal extracts of dandelion root contain the plant chemical inulin (not to be confused with the hormone insulin), which has a balancing effect on blood glucose levels. This can be used alongside the trace mineral chromium to help control fluctuating sugar levels associated with premenstrual problems.

Depression is suffered by about 30 per cent of women with PMS. This might be an effect of disordered brain chemistry (namely, serotonin) or a dysfunction of other brain chemicals. The exact cause is not known, but there appears to be a link with oestrogen levels. The extract from St. John's wort is very effective at relieving this type of depression. In one study, more than 65 per cent of those treated improved while using St. John's wort extract. The active agent, hypericin, was standardised in these tests.

It is not uncommon for women to gain more than 1.4kg (3lb), mostly due to water retention. The hormone to blame is aldosterone, which appears in excess in the premenstrual phase of the cycle, again linked to the oestrogen imbalance. A dose of uva-ursi taken from the time of ovulation (day 14 of the cycle) will increase the urine flow and control fluid retention.

The essential fatty acids contained in evening primrose oil can help with menstrual cramps and pain as well as help to balance hormone levels. A dose of 500–1,000mg taken at bedtime with water is recommended.

Substances such as feverfew extract have been able to stop prostaglandins from being produced, and this can be an important benefit for those who suffer menstrual discomfort.

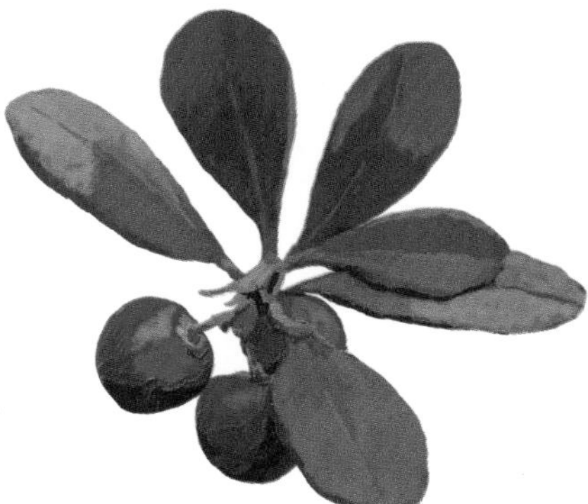

Uva-ursi can help to prevent pre-menstrual bloating.

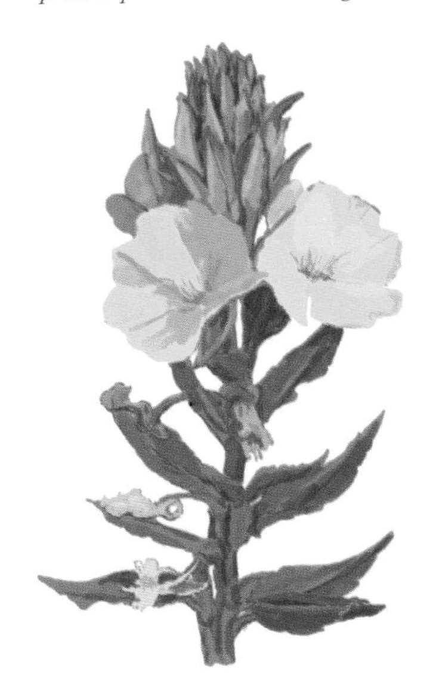

Oil of evening primrose can help with menstrual cramps.

CYSTITIS

Cystitis is generally caused by an infection travelling up from the vagina into the bladder. Flare-ups often occur after sexual intercourse, when the infection is reintroduced into the bladder.

Cystitis in men results from an infection travelling to the bladder from the urethra or from the prostate gland, which may itself be harbouring a bacterial infection. The most common symptoms in both men and women are pain and urgency – a constant sensation of the need to pass urine. Blood may be passed in the urine indicating the severity of the bladder infection. It is important to remember that the infection can travel up from the bladder into the kidneys and this complication requires urgent medical treatment.

Three-Step Treatment for Cystitis

Follow these simple steps for relief from cystitis.

Step 1 Increase your daily fluid intake to 2l (3½ pints) of water (preferably bottled water).

Step 2 Buy, or better still, make your own unsweetened cranberry juice and drink 500ml (18fl oz) daily. Cranberry powders and capsules are available. The dose for powders is 2 teaspoons taken in the morning and evening or two capsules taken twice daily. If you cannot obtain unsweetened cranberry juice, take the capsules or powders. Increasing your sugar intake by drinking sweetened cranberry juice will just encourage excessive bacterial growth in the bladder.

Step 3 Increase your general health and boost immunity by taking echinacea extract. Take 25–30 drops of liquid extract (or 2 capsules) twice daily.

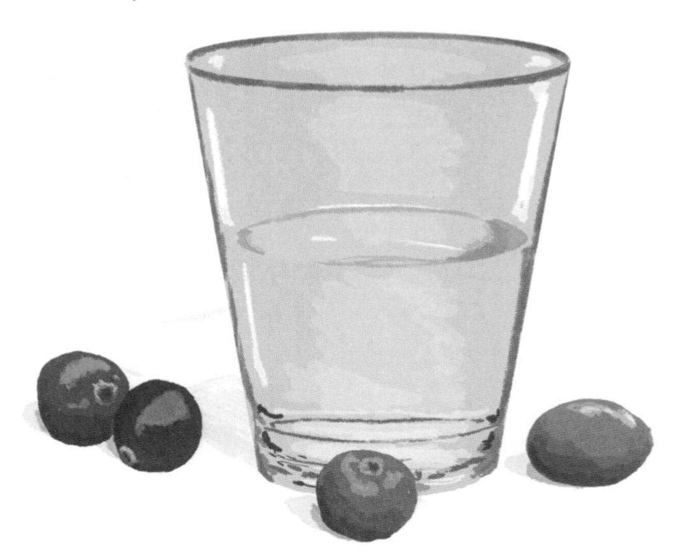

Drink more water and unsweetened cranberry juice for relief from cystitis.

IRRITABLE BOWEL SYNDROME (IBS)

The stomach and bowels are at work 24 hours a day digesting food, absorbing water and nutrients, killing invading bacteria and collecting waste matter. This activity needs to be controlled on a subconscious level, leaving the brain free to conduct day-to-day business.

In times of stress, the body brings the 'fight-or-flight' mechanism into play, releasing adrenaline and stimulating nervous activity. The bowel cannot contract and move normally and symptoms such as abdominal bloating, pain and cramping, fatigue, alternating bouts of constipation and diarrhoea, passage of mucus in the stool, flatulence and nausea are all common.

It is important to seek professional advice when bowel symptoms are experienced, since other conditions may mimic IBS – conditions such as lactose intolerance, coeliac disease, diverticular disease and bowel cancer. IBS needs an individual treatment programme, but some guidelines can be followed that may give relief.

Dietary Fibre Increasing the intake of soluble dietary fibre from vegetables, fruits, oat bran, beans and psyllium husk can be beneficial. However, this must be done slowly since the bowel in IBS tends to be hyperactive and may respond unfavourably to an unaccustomed dose of fibre.

Bowel Spasms For the symptomatic control of bowel spasms, try peppermint oil capsules, which have a relaxing effect on the smooth muscle that forms the bowel wall. Other antispasmodic agents are the herbs valerian, rosemary, chamomile and lemon balm.

Diarrhoea When diarrhoea and irritation are the main symptoms, an old preparation called Robert's formula has survived. It combines marshmallow root, cabbage extract, echinacea, goldenseal, okra and slippery elm. Modern preparations of Robert's formula are available in capsules and should be taken at a dose of 1 or 2 capsules between meals.

Nausea The nausea experienced by sufferers may be helped by taking ginger. Studies have documented how effective ginger can be in treating motion sickness and nausea. Ginger used in cooking or taken as a dietary supplement will not upset sensitive bowels, and it may calm the spastic nature of IBS as well as reduce the nausea.

Psychological Aspects The psychological aspects of IBS should not be overlooked. Almost all sufferers complain of fatigue, anxiety, depression, feelings of hostility, or sleep disturbances. These problems need attention and can be overcome with the correct help.

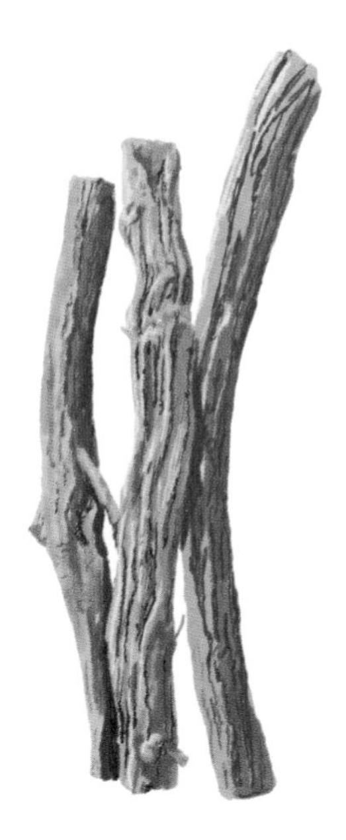

Licorice root

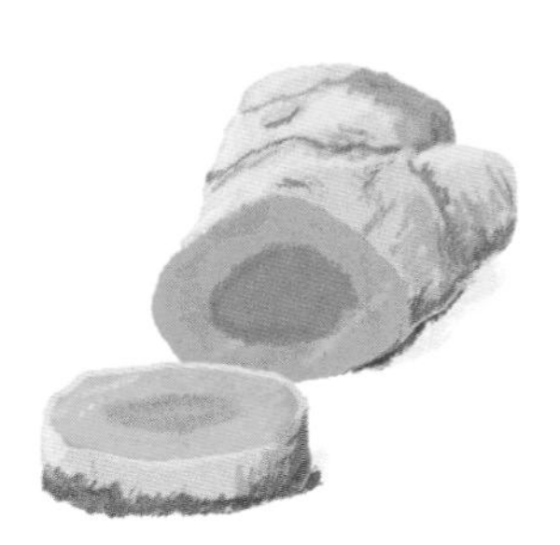

Turmeric

Pregnant and Breastfeeding Women

No pregnant woman should take any preparation without first consulting with her health-care practitioner. However, this – more than any other time – is a period when women often choose to turn to gentle herbal remedies over conventional medicines.

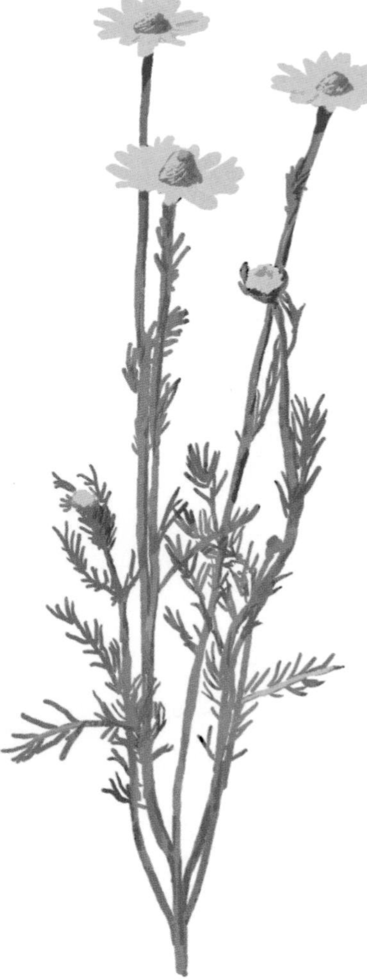

Chamomile tea makes a soothing drink before bedtime to help you to get a good night's sleep.

MORNING SICKNESS

No one knows the cause of morning sickness, but teas made from fennel, peppermint or ginger can give relief from symptoms. Taking a night-time cup of chamomile, lemon balm or hop tea will help you get a restful sleep.

There have been suggestions that ginger may be toxic during pregnancy, but all of the reviews state that the intake obtained via a tea is safe. The problem can arise when multiple concentrated extracts are taken in capsule or tablet form.

EMOTIONAL PROBLEMS

During pregnancy, moods may swing, and emotions become unbalanced. It is important to relax and have a good soak in a warm bath using a few drops of essential oils. Lavender and chamomile oil can be very relaxing. A tincture of rosemary can also help.

HEARTBURN

As the baby grows, it will take up a lot of space within your lower abdomen. This causes the stomach to become pushed up, and its contents occasionally leak into the lower part of the food pipe causing heartburn. Attention to diet is vital, as is taking digestive aids such as dill or caraway. These can be chewed or made into a tea and sipped during or between meals. Powdered slippery elm bark can give relief from the irritation of stomach acid.

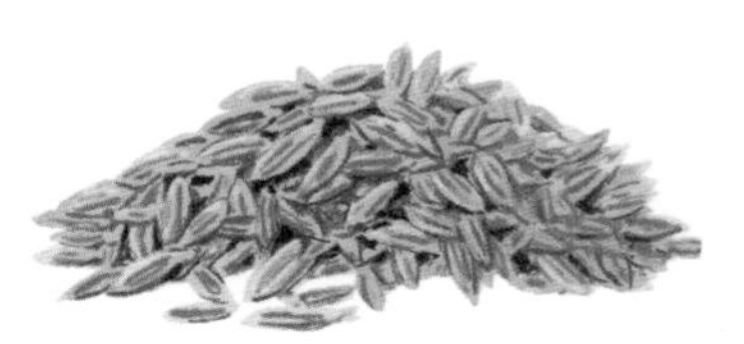

Caraway can aid digestion and help to ease or prevent heartburn.

VARICOSE VEINS AND HAEMORRHOIDS

To prevent these, you will need to include garlic in daily meals to keep the circulation strong. Try a tea made from dandelion. Extracts of St. John's wort can be made into a tea and taken two or three times daily.

To strengthen the walls of the veins and help to prevent bleeding, drink a tea made from fresh ginger. If the skin is irritated, try making a compress from comfrey and marshmallow.

For an intensive treatment of haemorrhoids that may be bleeding, apply a comfrey cream directly to the area.

Herbs to Avoid During Pregnancy

Mild herbal teas can bring relief from many pregnancy-related ailments, but you should not drink more than four cups a day. Oils and extracts contain higher doses of medicinal herbs and are best avoided during pregnancy, particularly those listed below.

- Yarrow (*Achillea millefolium*)
- Angelica (*Angelica archangelica*)
- Camomile (*Anthemis nobilis*)
- Celery (*Apium graveolens*)
- Bearberry (*Arctostaphylos uva-ursi*)
- Arnica (*Arnica montana*)
- Wormwood (*Artemisia absinthium*)
- Southernwood (*Artemisia abrotanum*)
- Calendula (*Calendula officinalis*)
- Gotu kola (*Centella asiatica*)
- Black cohosh (*Cimicifuga racemosa*)
- Myrrh (*Commiphora molmol*)
- Eyebright (*Euphrasis officinalis*)
- Fennel (*Foeniculum vulgare*)
- Licorice (*Glycyrrhiza glabra*)
- Goldenseal (*Hydrastis canadensis*)
- Hyssop (*Hyssopus officinalis*)
- Juniper (*Juniperus communis*)
- Devil's claw (*Martynia annua*)
- Nutmeg (*Myristica fragrans*)
- Pennyroyal (*Mentha pulegium*)
- Sweet marjoram (*Origanum majorana*)
- Parsley (*Petroselinum crispum*)
- Poke root (*Phytolacca americana*)
- Raspberry leaves (*Rubus idaeus*)
- Rye (*Ruta graveolens*)
- Sage (*Salvia officinalis*)
- Clary (*Salvia sclarea*)
- Feverfew (*Tanacetum parthenium*)
- Tansy (*Tanacetum vulgare*)
- Thuja (*Thuja occidentalis*)
- Thyme (*Thymus vulgaris*)
- Vervain (*Verbena officinalis*)

LACTATION

Remedies to encourage the flow of breast milk have been used for centuries. Infusions of milk thistle, nettle, fenugreek and hops are all safe to use and may also help to reduce the likelihood of colic in the baby.

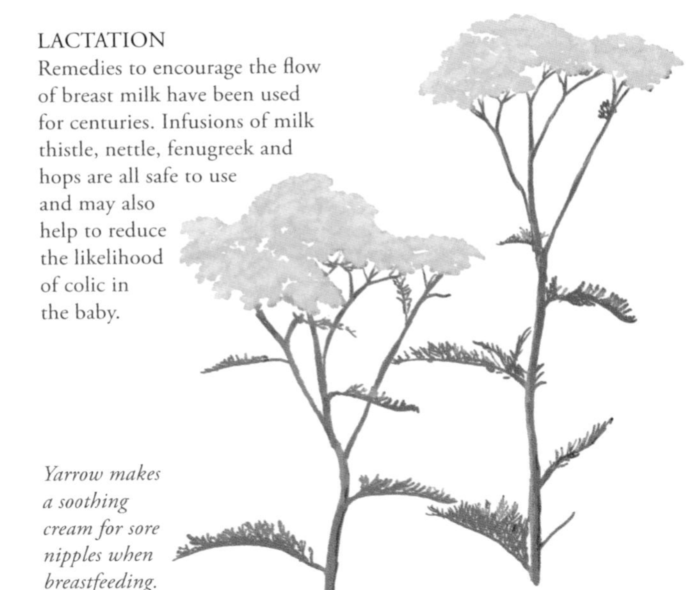

Yarrow makes a soothing cream for sore nipples when breastfeeding.

MASTITIS

If caught early, this condition can be reversed without antibiotics. As soon as mastitis is suspected, start expressing your milk, and take a dose of linseed oil, 1–3 tablespoons daily. If there is no improvement within 48 hours, seek medical advice.

SORE NIPPLES

The use of comfrey cream has been questioned by those who consider that accidental intake of the cream from the nipple when feeding the baby is dangerous. There is little evidence of risk, but if you wish to avoid this cream, use a yarrow-based cream instead. Do not use yarrow if you are pregnant.

Menopause Symptoms

It has been reported that up to 75 per cent of women suffer unpleasant menopause symptoms due to decreasing levels of hormones. For the majority, the symptoms may be short-term (lasting for two to three years), but for others they may persist for more than five years, making life intolerable.

Menopause symptoms are likely to occur at about 50 years of age, unless surgery (hysterectomy) brings on symptoms earlier. Menstruation usually becomes irregular until it stops altogether, emotions may alter, and the person may become more forgetful, and the sleep pattern could change, especially if night sweats are troublesome. Other symptoms may include hot flushes, joint stiffness, vaginal dryness, loss of sexual interest, anxiety, recurrent urinary tract infections, changes in hair, nail and skin quality, and loss of self-esteem.

Many of these problems are short-term, but other symptoms may not appear until much damage has been done. These include osteoporosis and the effects of heart disease and elevated blood cholesterol.

Food and plant extracts that have a phytoestrogen activity (an oestrogen-like activity but extracted from a plant) in the body can help to alleviate some symptoms. Foods naturally high in phytoestrogens include soy, fennel, celery, parsley, linseed oil, nuts and seeds.

Many herbs have been used in traditional folk medicine as uterine tonics, formulated to relieve menopause symptoms. The classic example is black cohosh, but licorice, chaste berry and ginseng are considered to be good sources as well.

Native Americans used black cohosh as a remedy for menstrual cramps and symptoms of menopause. Studies have concluded that the plant has a helpful oestrogen-like effect by virtue of its ability to rebalance hormone levels.

Panax ginseng (also known as Korean ginseng) was viewed as a masculine 'tonic' until its oestrogen-like activity was demonstrated. This action can be so strong that in high doses, the extract may induce postmenopausal bleeding.

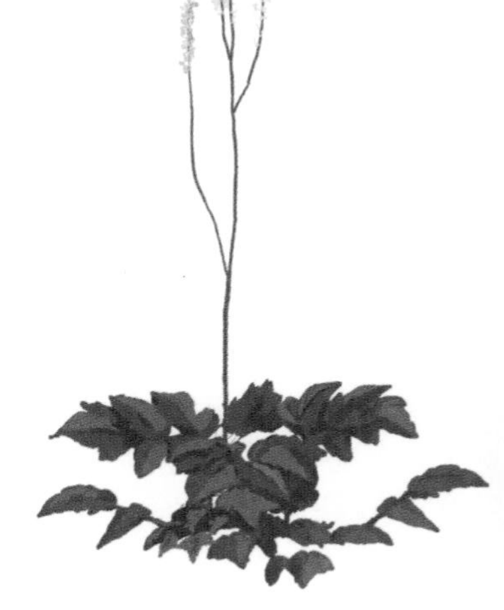

Black cohosh has a long history of use to treat menopause symptoms.

Formulas for Menopause

The following daily formulas are recommended as part of a natural treatment programme. Use one or the other.

Formula 1

- Licorice extract (*Glycyrrhiza glabra*) 25mg
- Black cohosh (*Cimicifuga racemosa*) 25mg
- Chaste berry extract (*Vitex anguscastus*) 25mg
- Fennel seed extract (*Foeniculum vulgare*) 12mg

Formula 2

- Vitamin E 150 IU
- Linseed oil (*Linum usitatissimum*) 300mg
- Gamma-oryzanol 100mg

The Elderly

One of the most common and debilitating conditions to affect the elderly is arthritis. There are many different types: some result in extreme inflammation and joint deformity; others cause long-term pain and stiffness. Herbal remedies can help to bring relief from most arthritic pain.

Osteoarthritis is the most common type of joint condition. The smooth joint coverings lose their ability to provide frictionless motion, causing degeneration of the joint. The cartilage starts to develop patches where its surface has become eroded. This acts as a focus for more erosion, and what was once a small patch soon expands into a much larger area of degeneration. The visible signs of arthritis are a thickening of the tissue and the appearance of nodules around the edges of the joint.

Natural diuretic herbs can help in the elimination of toxic substances such as uric acid by increasing the flow of urine. The two formulas listed (right) have a safe and effective action on the kidneys, and they are best combined with a special herbal tea, known as golden grass tea. To support the elimination process and assist in the reduction of inflammation, a combination herbal tincture remedy can be very effective.

Massage given by a qualified therapist can be a great relief when applied to the muscle structures that surround the degenerated joint. Massage increases circulation, aids in the drainage of tissue fluids, and stimulates the release of healing substances. Aromatherapy can also be helpful. Useful aromatherapy oils for arthritis include eucalyptus, ginger, lavender and rosemary.

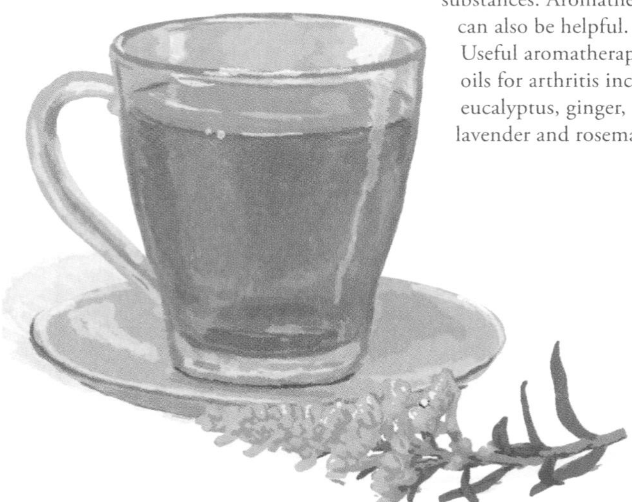

Formulas for Arthritis

Formula 1 (tincture)
- 50% Goldenrod (*Solidago virguaria*)
- 14% Silverweed (*Potentilla anserina*)
- 13% Birch (*Betula alba*)
- 5% *Ononis spinosa*
- 5% Pansy (*Viola tricolor*)
- 5% *Polygonum aviculare*
- 4% Horsetail (*Equisetum arvense*)
- 4% Juniper (*Juniperus communis*)

Formula 2 (solid extracts)
- Uva-ursi (*Arctostaphylos uva-ursi*) 100mg
- *Lespedeza capitatae* 50mg
- Boldo (*Peumus boldo*) 50mg
- Goldenrod (*Solidago virguaria*) 50mg

Golden Grass Tea
- 40% Goldenrod (*Solidago virguaria*)
- 30% *Betula alba*
- 15% Birch (*Polygonum avicularea*)
- 10% Horsetail (*Equisetum arvense*)
- 5% Pansy (*Viola tricolor*)

A tea of goldenrod can be mixed with formulas to treat arthritis.

COMMON PROBLEMS AND REMEDIES

It is recommended that you consult a health-care professional before embarking on a programme of self-treatment.

Alzheimer's Disease

- Tincture or capsules of ginkgo (*Ginkgo biloba)*

Angina

- Tincture or capsules of hawthorn (*Crataegus oxyacantha*)

Atherosclerosis

- Extract of garlic (*Allium sativum*)
- Extract of alfalfa (*Medicago sativa*
- Tincture or capsules of ginger (*Zingiber officinale*)

Bronchitis

- Extract of licorice (*Glycyrrhiza glabra*)
- Tincture of echinacea (*Echinacea purpura*)
- Extract of garlic (*Allium sativum*)

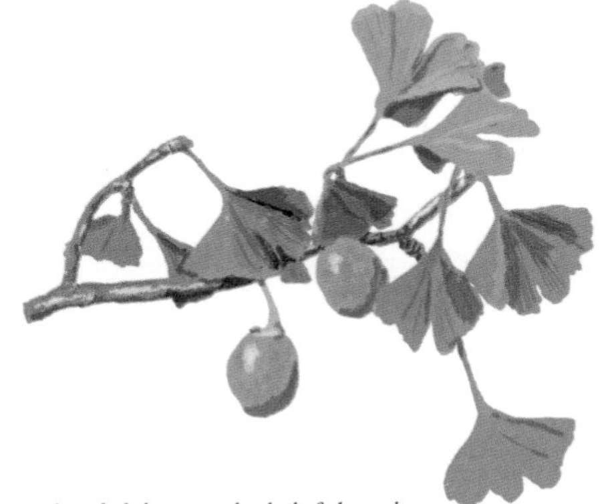

Ginkgo biloba may be helpful in the treatment of Alzheimer's disease.

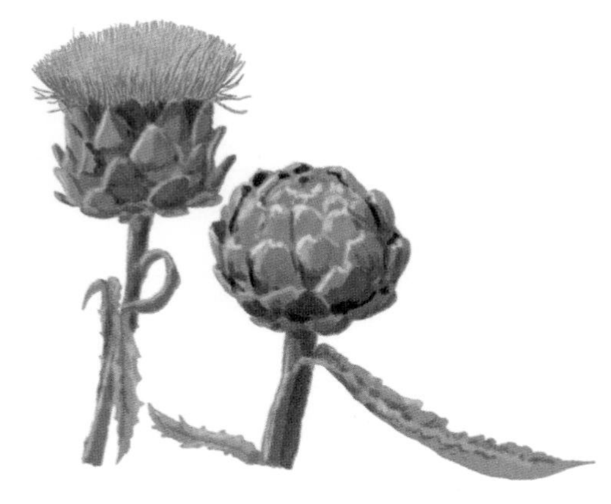

In some cases, an artichoke tincture can help to control diabetes.

Diabetes

- Extract of aloe vera (*Alo barbadensis*)
- Extract of bilberry (*Vaccinium myrtillus*)
- Extract of fenugreek (*Trigonella foenum-graecum*)
- Extract of garlic (*Allium sativum*)
- Tincture or capsules of ginkgo (*Ginkgo biloba*)
- Tincture of burdock (*Arctium lappa*)
- Tincture of dandelion (*Taraxacum officinalis*)
- Tincture of artichoke (*Cynara scolymus*)

Glaucoma

- Tincture or capsules of gingko (*Gingko biloba*)

Prostate Disease

- Tincture of nettle (*Urtica dioica*)

Varicose Veins

- Extract of bilberry (*Vaccinium myrtillus*)
- Tincture or capsules of ginkgo (*Ginkgo biloba*)
- Tincture of horse chestnut (*Aesculus hippocastanum*
- Tincture of hawthorn (*Crataegus oxyacantha*)

Remedies for Times of Stress

The symptoms of stress are different in us all, ranging from irritability and headaches to cold sores and more serious medical conditions, such as palpitations or high blood pressure. These herbal remedies can help to reduce your symptoms and treat an outbreak of cold sores.

There is no sign like an eruption of cold sores to indicate that the body is under stress. The immune system becomes suppressed, and opportunistic diseases such as *herpes simplex* make their appearance.

Lemon balm has been known as an herbal remedy for more than 2,000 years. During the 1960s, the dried extract was reported to exhibit antiviral activity in a number of studies. The efficiency of cream containing lemon balm depends on starting the therapy within eight hours of the onset of symptoms. And to be effective, the cream needs to be very concentrated, containing a 70:1 lemon balm extract with 1 per cent allantoin.

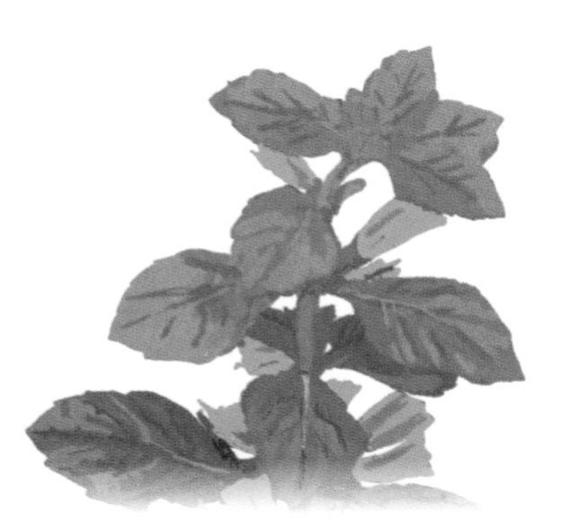

A lemon balm tincture can help to soothe irritability.

COMMON PROBLEMS AND REMEDIES

Exhaustion
- Tincture of oats (*Avena sativa*)
- Extract of ginseng (*Eleutherococcus senticosus*)

Fatigue
- Tincture or tablets of hyssop (*Hyssopus officinalis*)
- Extract of ginseng (*Eleutherococcus senticosus*)

Headache
- Tincture of valerian (*Valeriana officinalis*)
- Extract of butterbur (*Petasites hybridus*)

High Blood Pressure
- Tincture of mistletoe (*Viscum alba*)
- Extract of garlic (*Allium sativum*)

Insomnia
- Tincture of passionflower (*Passiflora incarnata*)
- Tincture or capsules of valerian (*Valeriana officinalis*)

Irritability
- Tincture of oats (*Avena sativa*)
- Tincture of lemon balm (*Melissa officinalis*)
- Tincture of hops (*Humulus lupulus*)
- Tincture of valerian (*Valeriana officinalis*)
- Tincture of passionflower (*Passiflora incarnata*)

Migraine
- Extract of butterbur (*Petasites hybridus*)
- Tincture of lemon balm (*Melissa officinalis*)

Palpitations
- Tincture of hawthorn (*Crataegus oxyacantha*)
- Tincture of passionflower (*Passiflora incarnata*)

Poor Memory
- Tincture or capsules of ginkgo (*Ginkgo biloba*)

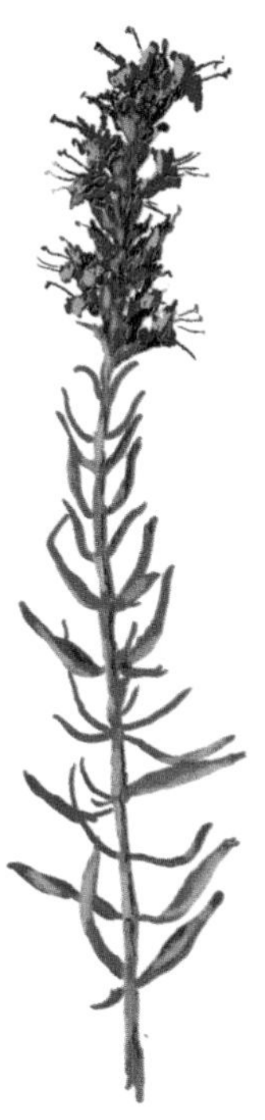

Hyssop is used to treat fatigue.

Emotional Problems

Depression, anxiety and panic attacks can affect all of us from time to time. It is estimated that nearly one in four people experiences some degree of depression at some time in their lives, with women tending to be at a slightly higher risk than men.

The biochemistry of mood disturbance is complex, but it is known that many nutritional and environmental factors play a vital role in psychological health.

An herbal substance that shows promise in the battle against depression is St. John's wort. This shrubby plant is native to Europe and has been used medicinally for centuries. Studies in Germany have found that the active agent, hypericin, alters brain chemistry and improves mood. Hypericin appears to be able to increase the brain's production of dopamine, an effect similar to many prescription drugs dispensed for depression.

Other studies have shown that a standardised extract of St. John's wort is more effective than prescription anti-depressants, such as amitriptyline, that are associated with significant side effects. The use of St. John's wort does not lead to any significant side effects.

St. John's wort preparations are available in 300mg capsules (standardised to contain 0.3% hypericin) and should be taken at the dose of two to three capsules daily.

Other herbs that may help in this condition include ginkgo and Siberian ginseng.

COMMON PROBLEMS AND REMEDIES

Anxiety

- Extract of kava kava (*Piper methysticum*), as needed
- Extract of Korean ginseng (*Panax ginseng*), as needed

Panic Attacks

- Valerian (*Valeriana officinalis*) capsules, as needed.

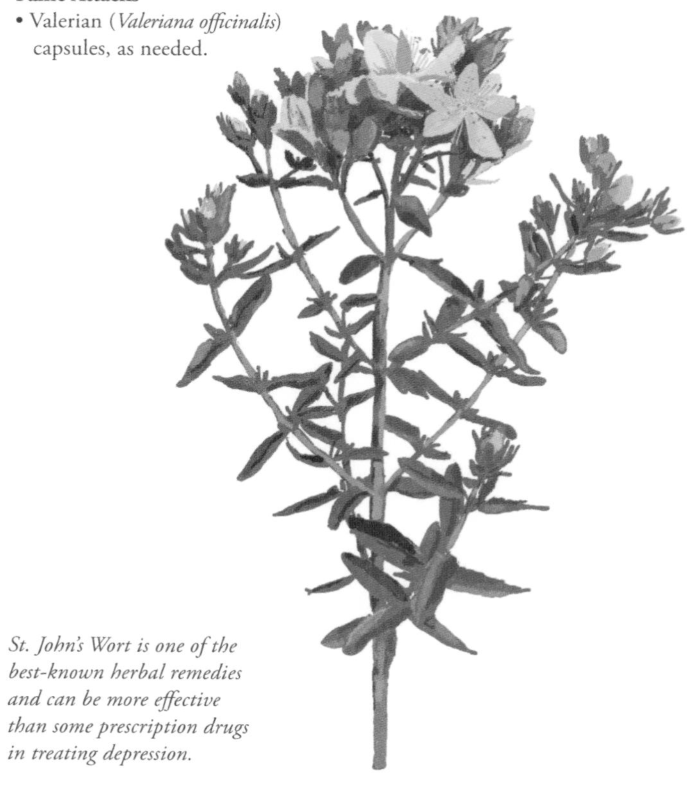

St. John's Wort is one of the best-known herbal remedies and can be more effective than some prescription drugs in treating depression.

Over-the-counter Remedies

Each remedy listed here will support and stimulate the itemised function or system, and in the case of vaginal thrush (*Candida albicans*), the aim is to eliminate the condition. All these remedies are readily available in pharmacies and health food shops.

Adrenal Function
- Korean ginseng (*Panax ginseng*)
- Siberian ginseng (*Eleutherococcus senticosus*)
- Licorice (*Glycyrrhiza glabra*)

Bladder Health
- Cranberry (*Vaccinium macrocarpon*)
- Uva-ursi (*Arctostaphylos uva-ursi*)

Bowel Function
- Fenugreek (*Trigonella foenum-graecum*)
- Ginger (*Zingiber officinale*)
- Marshmallow (*Althea officinalis*)
- Peppermint (*Mentha piperita*)

Eye Function
- Bilberry (*Vaccinium myrtillus*)

Heart and Circulation
- Cayenne pepper (*Capsicum frutescens*)
- Garlic (*Allium sativum*)
- Ginkgo (*Ginkgo biloba*)

Hormone (Female) Function
- Fennel seed (*Foeniculum vulgare*)
- Licorice (*Glycyrrhiza glabra*)

Hormone (Male) and Prostate Function
- Ginkgo (*Ginkgo biloba*)
- Korean ginseng (*Panax ginseng*)

Immune System
- Echinacea (*Echinacea purpura*)
- Goldenseal (*Hydrastis canadensis*)

Joints
- Butterbur (*Petasites hybridus*)
- Horsetail (*Equisetum arvense*)
- Peppermint (*Mentha piperita*)
- Yarrow (*Achillea millefolium*)

Kidney Function
- Uva-ursi extract (*Arctostaphylos uva-ursi*)
- Boldo extract (*Peumus boldo*)
- Goldenseal extract (*Hydrastis canadensis*)
- Horsetail (*Equisetum arvense*)
- Juniper (*Juniperus communis*)

Liver Function
- Boldo (*Peumus boldo*)
- Dandelion (*Taraxacum officinale*)
- Licorice (*Glycyrrhiza glabra*)
- Peppermint (*Mentha piperita*)

Lung Function
- Fenugreek (*Trigonella foenum-graecum*)
- Garlic (*Allium sativum*)
- Marshmallow (*Althaea officinalis*)
- Thyme (*Thymus vulgaris*)

Lymphatic System
- Goldenseal (*Hydrastis canadensis*)

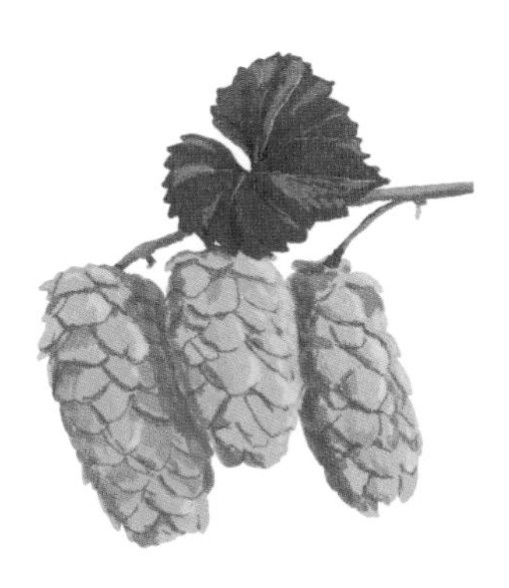

Hops may help to calm a troubled nervous system.

Nervous System
- Chamomile (*Anthemis nobilis*)
- Hops (*Humulus lupulus*)
- Passionflower (*Passiflora incarnata*)
- Valerian (*Valeriana officinalis*)

Skin Health
- Chamomile (*Anthemis nobilis*)
- Horsetail (*Equisetum arvense*)
- Rosemary (*Rosmarinus officinalis*)
- Sage (*Salvia officinalis*)

Vaginal Thrush
- Goldenseal (*Hydrastis canadensis*)
- Oregano (*Origanum vulgare*)
- Peppermint (*Mentha piperita*)
- Thyme (*Thymus vulgaris*)

Glossary

Addison's disease Disease caused by the underactivity of the adrenal glands

Adrenal glands Glands situated just above the kidneys

Adrenaline Hormone secreted by the adrenal gland that is released in response to physical and mental stress and initiates a variety of responses, including increasing the heart rate

Analgesic Relieves pain

Anaemia Deficiency of haemoglobin in the blood

Antiallergy Reduces allergic reactions

Antibacterial Prevents the formation of bacteria

Antibiotic Prevents the growth of bacteria

Anti-depressant Alleviates depression

Anti-inflammatory Reduces inflammation

Antimicrobial Destroys pathogenic microorganisms

Antiseptic Prevents the growth of bacteria

Antispasmodic Relieves muscle spasms or cramps

Aphrodisiac Increases sexual desire

Aromatherapy Therapeutic use of essential oils usually through massage

Bacteriostatic Prevents the growth of bacteria

Bitters Herbs that have a bitter taste that stimulate the appetite and aid digestion

Carminative Relieves flatulence and settles the digestive system

Cholagogic Stimulates the flow of bile into the intestine

Cicatrisant Promotes the healing of skin and formation of scar tissue

Colic Abdominal pain in the intestines

Cortisone-like action Reduces inflammation

Cystitis Painful inflammation of the bladder

Decongestant Helps eliminate nasal congestion

Diaphoretic Promotes sweating

Diuretic Stimulates the secretion of urine

Douche Application of liquid into the vagina

Dyspepsia Indigestion

Elixir Tincture with added sugar or syrup

Emmenagogue Stimulates menstruation

Essential oils Base materials in aromatherapy that are highly aromatic and volatile and are produced from plants by means of extraction, usually distillation

Expectorant Helps to expel mucus and relieves congestion in the digestive tract

Flatulence Large amounts of gas in the stomach and intestines

Flavonoid Substance responsible for the colours yellow and orange in herbs, fruit and vegetables

Histamine Substance released in response to allergic reactions

Holistic Approach that considers the patient's body, mind and spirit

Lactation Secretion of breast milk

Laxative Promotes the evacuation of the bowels

Mastitis Acute inflammation of the breasts

Mucilage Viscous liquid that forms a protective layer over the mucous membranes and skin

Nervine A nerve tonic that calms the nerves

Neuralgia Acute nerve pain

Osteoporosis Loss of bone tissue

Phlegm Mucus secreted by the respiratory tract

Pleurisy Inflammation of the pleural membrane that surrounds the lungs

Rhizome Underground rootlike structure used as a food store by plants during the winter

Saponin Substance that forms a lather when mixed with water that is found in a variety of herbs and has a wide range of therapeutic properties

Sedative Relieves nervousness and induces sleep with a calming effect

Serotonin Hormone released from the pituitary gland in the brain

Sinusitis Inflammation of the sinuses

Tonic Herbs to strengthen and invigorate a specific organ, system or the whole body

Volatile Evaporates very easily when exposed to air

Index

V

W

Y

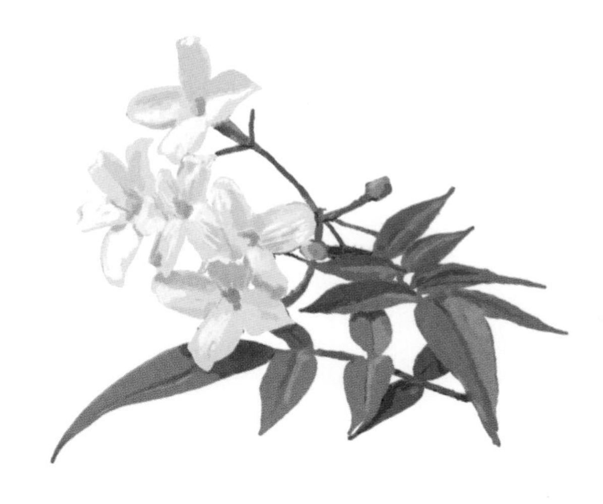